THIS KETO DIET

Journal Belongs To:

_____

KETO BEFORE & *After*

WEIGHT	WEIGHT
BMI	BMI
BODY FAT	BODY FAT
MUSCLE	MUSCLE
CHEST	CHEST
WAIST	WAIST
HIPS	HIPS
THIGHS	THIGHS
CALF	CALF
BICEP	BICEP
OTHER :	OTHER :
OTHER :	OTHER :

WEIGHT LOSS *Tracker*

MONTHLY GOAL

DATE:

BUST					
WAIST					
HIPS					
BICEP					
THIGH					
CALF					
WEIGHT					

TOTAL WEIGHT LOSS >>

MONTHLY PROGRESS *Tracker*

JAN   FEB   MAR   APR   MAY   JUN   JUL   AUG   SEP   OCT   NOV   DEC

MON	TUE	WED	THU	FRI	SAT	SUN

WEIGHT LOSS MILESTONE TRACKER

CHEAT DAY TRACKER

WEEKLY DIET SUCCESS TRACKER & NOTES

Keto 15 Task Challenge

1 CREATE A KETO JOURNAL AND DOCUMENT YOUR PROGRESS **COMPLETED** ☐	**2** CHOOSE 7 KETO FRIENDLY RECIPES TO TRY **COMPLETED** ☐	**3** CREATE A WEEKLY MEAL PLANNER **COMPLETED** ☐
4 LOG EVERYTHING YOU EAT IN A WEIGHT LOSS APP **COMPLETED** ☐	**5** PURCHASE A FOOD SCALE AND SPIRALIZER **COMPLETED** ☐	**6** TRY BULLET PROOF COFFEE **COMPLETED** ☐
7 WEIGH YOURSELF EVERY WEEK **COMPLETED** ☐	**8** GO ALCOHOL FREE FOR ONE WEEK **COMPLETED** ☐	**9** TRY A 12-HOUR INTERMITTENT FAST **COMPLETED** ☐
10 CHECK AND LOG YOUR BODY MEASUREMENTS **COMPLETED** ☐	**11** LIST ALL THE REASONS WHY KETO WILL WORK FOR YOU **COMPLETED** ☐	**12** LEARN TO MAKE FAT BOMBS **COMPLETED** ☐
13 MONITOR YOUR WATER INTAKE **COMPLETED** ☐	**14** INCREASE YOUR HEALTHY FAT INTAKE **COMPLETED** ☐	**15** TEST KETONE LEVELS USING STRIPS **COMPLETED** ☐

Ketogenic Foods

MEATS

Beef
Sausage
Bacon
Lamb
Pork
Veal
Chicken/Turkey
Eggs

VEGGIES

Avocado
Asparagus
Argula
Broccoli
Cauliflower
Brussel Sprouts
Cabbage
Celery

VEGGIES

Cucumber
Chards
Bell Peppers
Green Beans
Collards
Mushrooms
Spinach
Olives

FRUITS

Blackberries
Cranberries
Blueberries
Lemon
Lime
Raspberries
Strawberries
Plantains (paleo)

DAIRY

Cheese (all kinds)
Sour Cream
Cream Cheese
Heavy Cream
Greek Yogurt
Almond Milk
Cashew Milk
Coconut Cream

CONDIMENTS

Balsamic Vinegar
Beef/Chicken Broth
Bonito Flakes
Tartar Sauce (keto)
Dijon Mustard
Mayo
Low Sugar Ketchup
Pickles

OILS & FATS

Avocado Oil
Butter
Coconut Butter
Duck Fat
Lard/Ghee
Nut Oils
Olive Oil
Pork Rinds

HERBS & SPICES

Garlic
Salt & Pepper
Oregano
Paprika
Cumin
Chili Pepper
Basil
Ginger

BAKING

Almond Flour
Almond Meal
Cashew Flour
Oat Fiber
Psyllium Husk
Whey Protein
Flax meal
Hazelnut Flour

FISH/SEAFOOD

Anchovy
Haddock / Cod
Halibut
Crab/Lobster
Mackerel
Salmon
Tuna
Red Snapper

DRINKS

Diet Soda (moderation)
Coffee
Tea
Gatorade Zero
Protein Shake
Club Soda
Broth
Coconut Water

MISC.

Canned Tuna
Pesto
Soy Sauce
Aioli
Béarnaise
Vinaigrette
Hot Sauce
Guacamole

NOTES:

Yearly Keto Day Tracker

	JAN	FEB	MAR	APR	MAY	JUN	JUL	AUG	SEP	OCT	NOV	DEC
1												
2												
3												
4												
5												
6												
7												
8												
9												
10												
11												
12												
13												
14												
15												
16												
17												
18												
19												
20												
21												
22												
23												
24												
25												
26												
27												
28												
29												
30												
31												

COLOR IN THE DAYS THAT YOU WERE IN KETOSIS TO KEEP TRACK OF YOUR WEIGHT LOSS PROGRESS!

NOTES & REFLECTIONS:

TOTAL DAYS IN KETOSIS:

MONTH BY MONTH *Tracker*

JANUARY

JULY

FEBRUARY

AUGUST

MARCH

SEPTEMBER

APRIL

OCTOBER

MAY

NOVEMBER

JUNE

DECEMBER

MILESTONES

NOTES & REFLECTIONS

WEIGHT LOSS *Start Date*

Outline your most important fitness goals

Describe how you see yourself in six months

DATE   KETO WEIGHT LOSS ACTION PLAN   PERSONAL MILESTONES

WEIGHT LOSS *Journal*

MONDAY

TUESDAY

WEDNESDAY

THURSDAY

FRIDAY

SATURDAY

SUNDAY

WEEK OF:

DATE	WEIGHT LOSS ACTION PLAN

NOTES

MY WEIGHT LOSS *Routine*

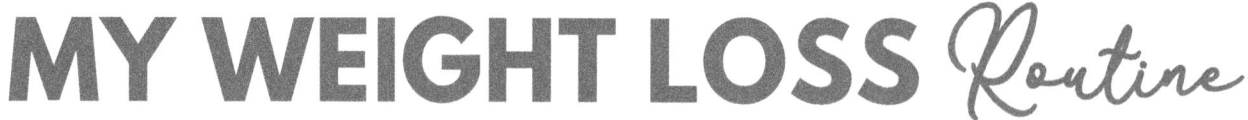

CREATING A ROUTINE FOR SUCCESS

WEIGHT LOSS SUCCESS: HABIT & ROUTINE TRACKER	
DRINK LOTS OF WATER TODAY	TRACK TOTAL CARB INTAKE

COMPLETE TOP 3 GOALS OF THE DAY

1
2
3

PLAN MY MEALS FOR THE DAY:

BREAKFAST	LUNCH	DINNER

DAILY TRACKER & TO DO LIST	ACCOMPLISHMENTS

NOTES

MY KETO *Routine*

Morning	My Weight Loss Routine	m t w t f s s

Mid Day	My Weight Loss Routine	m t w t f s s

Evening	My Weight Loss Routine	m t w t f s s

Night	My Weight Loss Routine	m t w t f s s

WEEKLY *Fasting Tracker*

Week Of: _____

MONDAY

Goal	12	1	2	3	4	5	6	7	8	9	10	11	12	1	2	3	4	5	6	7	8	9	10	11
Actual	12	1	2	3	4	5	6	7	8	9	10	11	12	1	2	3	4	5	6	7	8	9	10	11

TUESDAY

Goal	12	1	2	3	4	5	6	7	8	9	10	11	12	1	2	3	4	5	6	7	8	9	10	11
Actual	12	1	2	3	4	5	6	7	8	9	10	11	12	1	2	3	4	5	6	7	8	9	10	11

WEDNESDAY

Goal	12	1	2	3	4	5	6	7	8	9	10	11	12	1	2	3	4	5	6	7	8	9	10	11
Actual	12	1	2	3	4	5	6	7	8	9	10	11	12	1	2	3	4	5	6	7	8	9	10	11

THURSDAY

Goal	12	1	2	3	4	5	6	7	8	9	10	11	12	1	2	3	4	5	6	7	8	9	10	11
Actual	12	1	2	3	4	5	6	7	8	9	10	11	12	1	2	3	4	5	6	7	8	9	10	11

FRIDAY

Goal	12	1	2	3	4	5	6	7	8	9	10	11	12	1	2	3	4	5	6	7	8	9	10	11
Actual	12	1	2	3	4	5	6	7	8	9	10	11	12	1	2	3	4	5	6	7	8	9	10	11

SATURDAY

Goal	12	1	2	3	4	5	6	7	8	9	10	11	12	1	2	3	4	5	6	7	8	9	10	11
Actual	12	1	2	3	4	5	6	7	8	9	10	11	12	1	2	3	4	5	6	7	8	9	10	11

SUNDAY

Goal	12	1	2	3	4	5	6	7	8	9	10	11	12	1	2	3	4	5	6	7	8	9	10	11
Actual	12	1	2	3	4	5	6	7	8	9	10	11	12	1	2	3	4	5	6	7	8	9	10	11

WEEKLY *Progress*

WEEK OF : _____

Monday

Tuesday

Wednesday

Thursday

Friday

Saturday

Sunday

Notes

WEEK OF:

KETO *Meal* LOG BOOK

	BREAKFAST	LUNCH	DINNER	SNACKS
MONDAY				
TUESDAY				
WEDNESDAY				
THURSDAY				
FRIDAY				
SATURDAY				
SUNDAY				

MY PROGRESS *Tracker*

SLEEP TRACKER: **DATE** _____

☀ | RISE: | 🌙 zᶻᶻ | BEDTIME: | 💭zᶻᶻ | SLEEP (HRS): |

NOTES FOR THE DAY

_____
_____
_____

EXERCISE / WORKOUT ROUTINE

IN A STATE OF KETOSIS?

YES   NO   UNSURE

WATER INTAKE TRACKER

DAILY ENERGY LEVEL		
HIGH	**MEDIUM**	**LOW**

BREAKFAST

FAT: CARBS: PROTEIN: CALORIES:

LUNCH

FAT: CARBS: PROTEIN: CALORIES:

DINNER

FAT: CARBS: PROTEIN: CALORIES:

SNACKS

FAT: CARBS: PROTEIN: CALORIES:

TOP 6 PRIORITIES OF THE DAY

END OF THE DAY TOTAL OVERVIEW

CARBS	FAT	PROTEIN	CALORIES

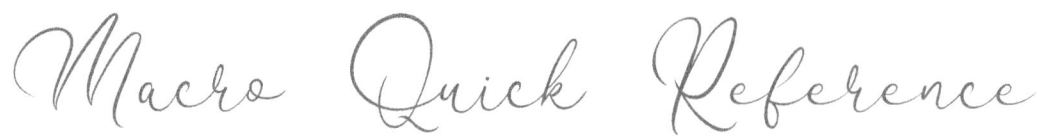

Macro Quick Reference

MACRO TRACKER

QTY	TYPE	PROTEIN	FAT	CARBS	CALS	NOTES

INTERMITTENT *Fasting Log*

WEEK OF:

	START TIME	END TIME	TOTAL FAST HRS
M	:	:	:
T	:	:	:
W	:	:	:
T	:	:	:
F	:	:	:
S	:	:	:
S	:	:	:

WEEK OF:

	START TIME	END TIME	TOTAL FAST HRS
M	:	:	:
T	:	:	:
W	:	:	:
T	:	:	:
F	:	:	:
S	:	:	:
S	:	:	:

WEEK OF:

	START TIME	END TIME	TOTAL FAST HRS
M	:	:	:
T	:	:	:
W	:	:	:
T	:	:	:
F	:	:	:
S	:	:	:
S	:	:	:

WEEK OF:

	START TIME	END TIME	TOTAL FAST HRS
M	:	:	:
T	:	:	:
W	:	:	:
T	:	:	:
F	:	:	:
S	:	:	:
S	:	:	:

WEEK OF:

	START TIME	END TIME	TOTAL FAST HRS
M	:	:	:
T	:	:	:
W	:	:	:
T	:	:	:
F	:	:	:
S	:	:	:
S	:	:	:

WEEK OF:

	START TIME	END TIME	TOTAL FAST HRS
M	:	:	:
T	:	:	:
W	:	:	:
T	:	:	:
F	:	:	:
S	:	:	:
S	:	:	:

MILESTONES & ACCOMPLISHMENTS

NOTES & REFLECTIONS

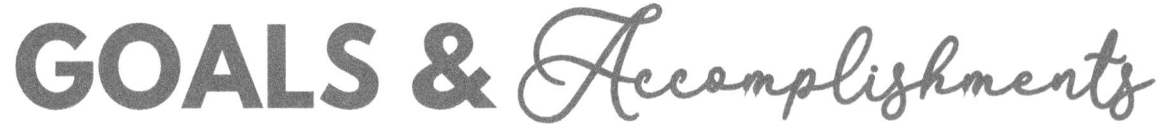

GOALS & *Accomplishments*

Month   JAN   FEB   MAR   APR   MAY   JUN   JUL   AUG   SEP   OCT   NOV   DEC

THIS MONTH'S **GOALS**

ACTION PLAN

M T W T F S S

☐☐☐☐☐☐☐
☐☐☐☐☐☐☐
☐☐☐☐☐☐☐
☐☐☐☐☐☐☐
☐☐☐☐☐☐☐

NOTES:

WEEKLY GOALS

M
T
W
T
F
S
S

THOUGHTS

MEALS:	BREAKFAST	LUNCH	DINNER	SNACKS
M				
T				
W				
T				
F				
S				
S				

Low Carb Grocery Ideas

FRESH PRODUCE

☐ Asparagus	☐ Cauliflower	☐ Onions
☐ Avocado	☐ Celery	☐ Radishes
☐ Bell Peppers	☐ Cucumber	☐ Salad Mix
☐ Berries	☐ Eggplant	☐ Squash
☐ Broccoli	☐ Fennel	☐ Tomatoes
☐ Brussel Sprouts	☐ Garlic	☐ Bok Choi
☐ Cabbage	☐ Green Beans	☐ Chives
☐ Carrots	☐ Mushrooms	☐ Spinach

MEAT AND SEAFOOD

☐ Bacon	☐ Lamb	☐ Fish
☐ Beef	☐ Pork	☐ Crab
☐ Bison	☐ Rotisserie Chicken	☐ Lobster
☐ Chicken	☐ Sausage	☐ Scallops
☐ Deli meat	☐ Turkey	☐ Shrimp
☐ Ground Beef / Ground Turkey	☐ Oyster	☐ Mussels

DAIRY PRODUCTS

☐ Butter	☐ Eggs	☐ Sour Cream
☐ Cheese	☐ Greek Yogurt, full fat	☐ Ghee
☐ Cream Cheese	☐ Heavy Whipping Cream	☐ Mayo

PANTRY ITEMS

☐ Avocado oil	☐ Tea/Coffee	☐ Moon Cheese
☐ Beef Jerky	☐ Pork Rinds	☐ Low Carb Protein Bars
☐ Bone Broth	☐ Mayonnaise	☐ All Natural Peanut Butter
☐ Tuna, Salmon (canned)	☐ Low Carb Salad Dressing	☐ Stevia
☐ Coconut Butter	☐ Olive oil, extra virgin	☐ Almonds
☐ Coconut Oil	☐ Olives	☐ Spices
☐ Almond Milk	☐ Sweeteners	☐ Almond Flour

FROZEN / OTHER

☐	☐	☐
☐	☐	☐
☐	☐	☐
☐	☐	☐

Low Carb Shopping List

FRESH PRODUCE

MEAT AND SEAFOOD

DAIRY PRODUCTS

PANTRY ITEMS

FROZEN / OTHER

Keto Friendly Foods

KETO FRIENDLY FOODS	NET CARBS	PROTEINS	FAT

FOODS TO EAT IN MODERATION	NET CARBS	PROTEINS	FAT

STAYING *On Track*

MY WEIGHT LOSS DIARY:

WATER TRACKER

NOTES & REMINDERS

DOODLE MY MOOD

LOW CARB SNACKS

BREAKFAST IDEAS

LUNCH IDEAS

DINNER IDEAS

STAYING *On Track*

MY WEIGHT LOSS DIARY:

_____

_____

_____

_____

WATER TRACKER

LOW CARB SNACKS

NOTES & REMINDERS

DOODLE MY MOOD

BREAKFAST IDEAS

LUNCH IDEAS

DINNER IDEAS

STAYING *On Track*

MY WEIGHT LOSS DIARY:

WATER TRACKER

NOTES & REMINDERS

DOODLE MY MOOD

LOW CARB SNACKS

BREAKFAST IDEAS

LUNCH IDEAS

DINNER IDEAS

STAYING *On Track*

MY WEIGHT LOSS DIARY:

_____

_____

_____

_____

WATER TRACKER

NOTES & REMINDERS

DOODLE MY MOOD

LOW CARB SNACKS

BREAKFAST IDEAS

LUNCH IDEAS

DINNER IDEAS

STAYING *On Track*

MY WEIGHT LOSS DIARY:

WATER TRACKER

LOW CARB SNACKS

NOTES & REMINDERS

DOODLE MY MOOD

BREAKFAST IDEAS

LUNCH IDEAS

DINNER IDEAS

STAYING *On Track*

MY WEIGHT LOSS DIARY:

_____

_____

_____

_____

WATER TRACKER

◇ ◇ ◇ ◇ ◇ ◇ ◇ ◇

LOW CARB SNACKS

NOTES & REMINDERS

DOODLE MY MOOD

BREAKFAST IDEAS

LUNCH IDEAS

DINNER IDEAS

STAYING *On Track*

MY WEIGHT LOSS DIARY:

WATER TRACKER

NOTES & REMINDERS

DOODLE MY MOOD

LOW CARB SNACKS

BREAKFAST IDEAS

LUNCH IDEAS

DINNER IDEAS

MEAL *Planner*

GROCERY LIST

MON

TUES

WED

THUR

FRI

SAT

SUN

KETO *Recipe*

RECIPE NAME:

	Keto	Low Carb	Paleo	Vegetarian	Vegan	Dairy Free	Gluten Free
	☐	☐	☐	☐	☐	☐	☐

QTY	INGREDIENTS	RECIPE INSTRUCTIONS

NOTES & RECIPE REVIEW	
	Serves
	Prep Time
	Cook Time
	Tools
	Temp

Total	Carbs	Fat	Protein	Cals

DAILY FOOD *Tracker*

FOOD TRACKER

MEAL/SNACK	NET CARBS	FAT	CAL	PROTEIN
DAILY GOAL:				
TOTAL:				

NOTES & MEAL IDEAS

FITNESS TRACKER

Type		Notes
Time		
Avg HR		
Max HR		
Reps		
Cals		

DAILY OVERVIEW

Sleep		Notes		On Track
Water Intake				
Steps Taken				
Active Mins				Goal Met
Active Hours				
Cals Burned				

DAILY FOOD *Tracker*

FOOD TRACKER

MEAL/SNACK	NET CARBS	FAT	CAL	PROTEIN
DAILY GOAL:				
TOTAL:				

NOTES & MEAL IDEAS

FITNESS TRACKER

Type		Notes
Time		
Avg HR		
Max HR		
Reps		
Cals		

DAILY OVERVIEW

Sleep		Notes
Water Intake		
Steps Taken		
Active Mins		
Active Hours		
Cals Burned		

On Track

Goal Met

DAILY FOOD *Tracker*

FOOD TRACKER

MEAL/SNACK	NET CARBS	FAT	CAL	PROTEIN
DAILY GOAL:				
TOTAL:				

NOTES & MEAL IDEAS

FITNESS TRACKER

Type		Notes
Time		
Avg HR		
Max HR		
Reps		
Cals		

DAILY OVERVIEW

Sleep		Notes
Water Intake		
Steps Taken		
Active Mins		
Active Hours		
Cals Burned		

On Track

Goal Met

DAILY FOOD *Tracker*

FOOD TRACKER

MEAL/SNACK	NET CARBS	FAT	CAL	PROTEIN
DAILY GOAL:				
TOTAL:				

NOTES & MEAL IDEAS

FITNESS TRACKER

Type		Notes
Time		
Avg HR		
Max HR		
Reps		
Cals		

DAILY OVERVIEW

Sleep		Notes		On Track
Water Intake				
Steps Taken				
Active Mins				Goal Met
Active Hours				
Cals Burned				

DAILY FOOD *Tracker*

FOOD TRACKER

MEAL/SNACK	NET CARBS	FAT	CAL	PROTEIN
DAILY GOAL:				
TOTAL:				

NOTES & MEAL IDEAS

FITNESS TRACKER

		Notes
Type		
Time		
Avg HR		
Max HR		
Reps		
Cals		

DAILY OVERVIEW

		Notes		
Sleep			On Track	
Water Intake				
Steps Taken				
Active Mins			Goal Met	
Active Hours				
Cals Burned				

DAILY FOOD *Tracker*

FOOD TRACKER

MEAL/SNACK	NET CARBS	FAT	CAL	PROTEIN

DAILY GOAL:

TOTAL:

NOTES & MEAL IDEAS

FITNESS TRACKER

Type		Notes
Time		
Avg HR		
Max HR		
Reps		
Cals		

DAILY OVERVIEW

Sleep		Notes		On Track
Water Intake				
Steps Taken				
Active Mins				Goal Met
Active Hours				
Cals Burned				

DAILY FOOD *Tracker*

FOOD TRACKER

MEAL/SNACK	NET CARBS	FAT	CAL	PROTEIN
DAILY GOAL:				
TOTAL:				

NOTES & MEAL IDEAS

FITNESS TRACKER

		Notes
Type		
Time		
Avg HR		
Max HR		
Reps		
Cals		

DAILY OVERVIEW

		Notes		
Sleep			On Track	
Water Intake				
Steps Taken				
Active Mins			Goal Met	
Active Hours				
Cals Burned				

KETO GO TO *Meals*

FAVORITE KETO FRIENDLY MEALS

BREAKFAST	LUNCH	DINNER	SNACKS
BREAKFAST	LUNCH	DINNER	SNACKS
BREAKFAST	LUNCH	DINNER	SNACKS
BREAKFAST	LUNCH	DINNER	SNACKS
BREAKFAST	LUNCH	DINNER	SNACKS
BREAKFAST	LUNCH	DINNER	SNACKS
BREAKFAST	LUNCH	DINNER	SNACKS

12 WEEK *Keto Meal Tracker*

12 Week Keto Challenge

MONTH	JAN	FEB	MAR	APR	MAY	JUN	JUL	AUG	SEP	OCT	NOV	DEC
WEEK	01	02	03	04	05	06	07	08	09	10	11	12

	BREAKFAST	LUNCH	DINNER	SNACKS
M				
T				
W				
T				
F				
S				
S				

GROCERY SHOPPING LIST / RECIPE INGREDIENTS

Weekly Meal Planner

Week of: _____

	Breakfast	Lunch	Dinner	Snack	Other
Monday	TOTAL Carbs Fat Protein Cals	TOTAL Carbs Fat Protein Cals	TOTAL Carbs Fat Protein Cals	TOTAL Carbs Fat Protein Cals	TOTAL Carbs Fat Protein Cals
Tuesday	TOTAL Carbs Fat Protein Cals	TOTAL Carbs Fat Protein Cals	TOTAL Carbs Fat Protein Cals	TOTAL Carbs Fat Protein Cals	TOTAL Carbs Fat Protein Cals
Wednesday	TOTAL Carbs Fat Protein Cals	TOTAL Carbs Fat Protein Cals	TOTAL Carbs Fat Protein Cals	TOTAL Carbs Fat Protein Cals	TOTAL Carbs Fat Protein Cals
Thursday	TOTAL Carbs Fat Protein Cals	TOTAL Carbs Fat Protein Cals	TOTAL Carbs Fat Protein Cals	TOTAL Carbs Fat Protein Cals	TOTAL Carbs Fat Protein Cals
Friday	TOTAL Carbs Fat Protein Cals	TOTAL Carbs Fat Protein Cals	TOTAL Carbs Fat Protein Cals	TOTAL Carbs Fat Protein Cals	TOTAL Carbs Fat Protein Cals
Saturday	TOTAL Carbs Fat Protein Cals	TOTAL Carbs Fat Protein Cals	TOTAL Carbs Fat Protein Cals	TOTAL Carbs Fat Protein Cals	TOTAL Carbs Fat Protein Cals
Sunday	TOTAL Carbs Fat Protein Cals	TOTAL Carbs Fat Protein Cals	TOTAL Carbs Fat Protein Cals	TOTAL Carbs Fat Protein Cals	TOTAL Carbs Fat Protein Cals

100 Days of Keto

STARTING WEIGHT:	DAY 100 WEIGHT:

| 1 | 2 | 3 | 4 | 5 | 6 | 7 | 8 | 9 | 10 | LBS LOST:
INCHES LOST: |

| 11 | 12 | 13 | 14 | 15 | 16 | 17 | 18 | 19 | 20 | LBS LOST:
INCHES LOST: |

| 21 | 22 | 23 | 24 | 25 | 26 | 27 | 28 | 29 | 30 | LBS LOST:
INCHES LOST: |

| 31 | 32 | 33 | 34 | 35 | 36 | 37 | 38 | 39 | 40 | LBS LOST:
INCHES LOST: |

| 41 | 42 | 43 | 44 | 45 | 46 | 47 | 48 | 49 | 50 | LBS LOST:
INCHES LOST: |

| 51 | 52 | 53 | 54 | 55 | 56 | 57 | 58 | 59 | 60 | LBS LOST:
INCHES LOST: |

| 61 | 62 | 63 | 64 | 65 | 66 | 67 | 68 | 69 | 70 | LBS LOST:
INCHES LOST: |

| 71 | 72 | 73 | 74 | 75 | 76 | 77 | 78 | 79 | 80 | LBS LOST:
INCHES LOST: |

| 81 | 82 | 83 | 84 | 85 | 86 | 87 | 88 | 89 | 90 | LBS LOST:
INCHES LOST: |

| 91 | 92 | 93 | 94 | 95 | 96 | 97 | 98 | 99 | 100 | LBS LOST:
INCHES LOST: |

TOTAL WEIGHT LOST:	TOTAL INCHES LOST:

NOTES & REFLECTIONS:

24 DAY *Weight Loss Steps*

WEIGHT LOSS PLAN OF ACTION:

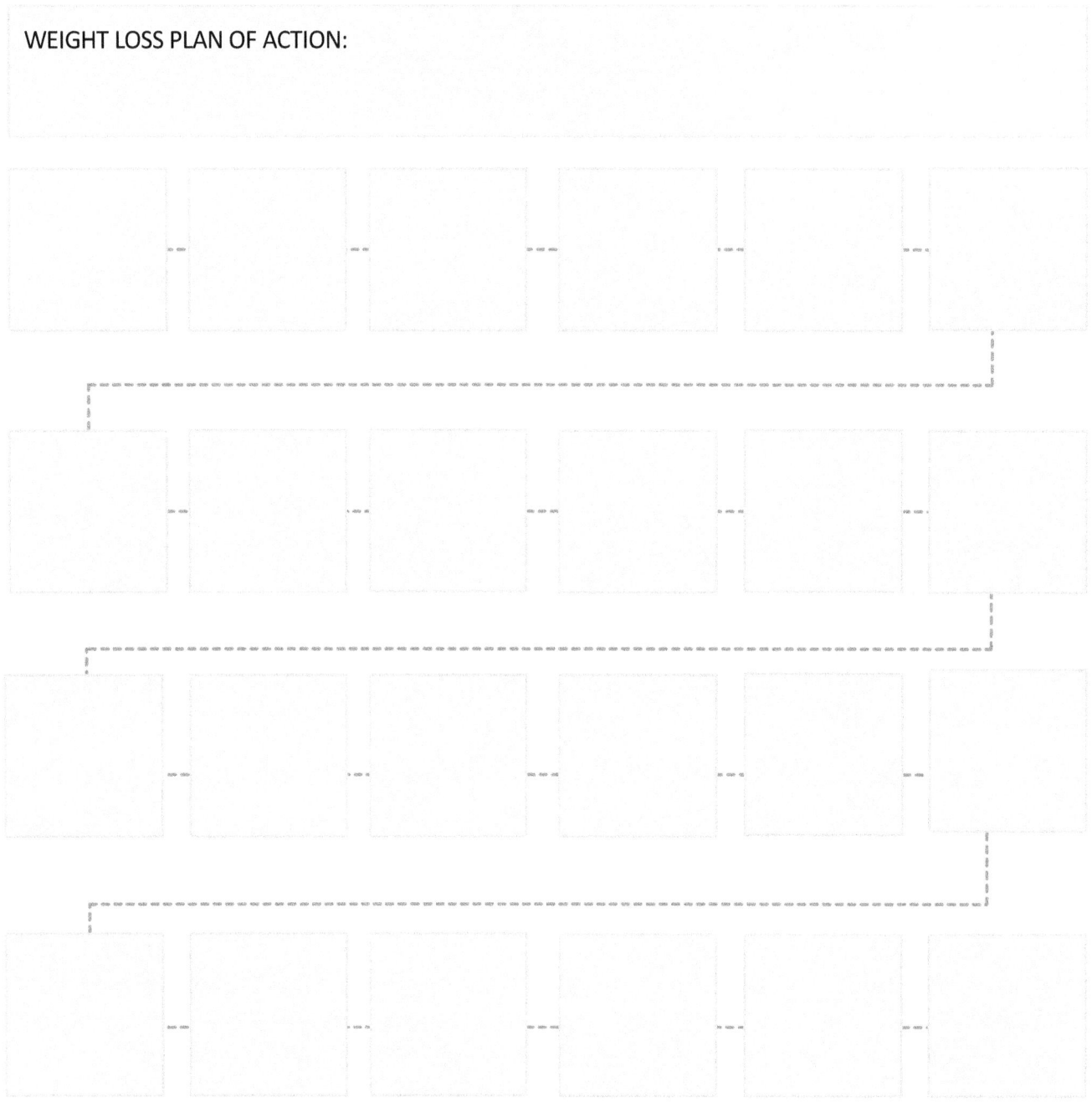

PERSONAL ACCOMPLISHMENTS

30 DAY *Keto Challenge*

MY PLAN OF ACTION

- [ ] _____
- [ ] _____
- [ ] _____
- [ ] _____
- [ ] _____
- [ ] _____
- [ ] _____
- [ ] _____
- [ ] _____
- [ ] _____
- [ ] _____
- [ ] _____
- [ ] _____
- [ ] _____
- [ ] _____
- [ ] _____

INSPIRATIONAL REMINDERS

_____
_____
_____
_____
_____
_____
_____

STARTED >

FINISHED >

1	2	3	4	5	6	7	8	9	10
11	12	13	14	15	16	17	18	19	20
21	22	23	24	25	26	27	28	29	30

30-DAY KETO RESULTS

PERSONAL ACCOMPLISHMENTS

60 Days of Keto

STARTING WEIGHT: _____   DAY 60 WEIGHT: _____

| 1 | 2 | 3 | 4 | 5 | 6 | 7 | 8 | 9 | 10 |

LBS LOST:
INCHES LOST:

| 11 | 12 | 13 | 14 | 15 | 16 | 17 | 18 | 19 | 20 |

LBS LOST:
INCHES LOST:

| 21 | 22 | 23 | 24 | 25 | 26 | 27 | 28 | 29 | 30 |

LBS LOST:
INCHES LOST:

| 31 | 32 | 33 | 34 | 35 | 36 | 37 | 38 | 39 | 40 |

LBS LOST:
INCHES LOST:

| 41 | 42 | 43 | 44 | 45 | 46 | 47 | 48 | 49 | 50 |

LBS LOST:
INCHES LOST:

| 51 | 52 | 53 | 54 | 55 | 56 | 57 | 58 | 59 | 60 |

LBS LOST:
INCHES LOST:

TOTAL WEIGHT LOST: _____   TOTAL INCHES LOST: _____

NOTES & REFLECTIONS:

30 Days of Keto

STARTING WEIGHT:

DAY 30 WEIGHT:

| 1 | 2 | 3 | 4 | 5 | 6 | 7 | 8 | 9 | 10 |

LBS LOST:
INCHES LOST:

| 11 | 12 | 13 | 14 | 15 | 16 | 17 | 18 | 19 | 20 |

LBS LOST:
INCHES LOST:

| 21 | 22 | 23 | 24 | 25 | 26 | 27 | 28 | 29 | 30 |

LBS LOST:
INCHES LOST:

TOTAL WEIGHT LOST:

TOTAL INCHES LOST:

NOTES:

PERSONAL ACCOMPLISHMENTS:

THOUGHTS & REFLECTIONS:

WEIGHT LOSS *Journal*

MONDAY

TUESDAY

WEDNESDAY

THURSDAY

FRIDAY

SATURDAY

SUNDAY

WEEK OF:

DATE	WEIGHT LOSS ACTION PLAN

NOTES

WEEKLY *Fasting Tracker*

Week Of: _____

MONDAY

Goal	12	1	2	3	4	5	6	7	8	9	10	11	12	1	2	3	4	5	6	7	8	9	10	11
Actual	12	1	2	3	4	5	6	7	8	9	10	11	12	1	2	3	4	5	6	7	8	9	10	11

TUESDAY

Goal	12	1	2	3	4	5	6	7	8	9	10	11	12	1	2	3	4	5	6	7	8	9	10	11
Actual	12	1	2	3	4	5	6	7	8	9	10	11	12	1	2	3	4	5	6	7	8	9	10	11

WEDNESDAY

Goal	12	1	2	3	4	5	6	7	8	9	10	11	12	1	2	3	4	5	6	7	8	9	10	11
Actual	12	1	2	3	4	5	6	7	8	9	10	11	12	1	2	3	4	5	6	7	8	9	10	11

THURSDAY

Goal	12	1	2	3	4	5	6	7	8	9	10	11	12	1	2	3	4	5	6	7	8	9	10	11
Actual	12	1	2	3	4	5	6	7	8	9	10	11	12	1	2	3	4	5	6	7	8	9	10	11

FRIDAY

Goal	12	1	2	3	4	5	6	7	8	9	10	11	12	1	2	3	4	5	6	7	8	9	10	11
Actual	12	1	2	3	4	5	6	7	8	9	10	11	12	1	2	3	4	5	6	7	8	9	10	11

SATURDAY

Goal	12	1	2	3	4	5	6	7	8	9	10	11	12	1	2	3	4	5	6	7	8	9	10	11
Actual	12	1	2	3	4	5	6	7	8	9	10	11	12	1	2	3	4	5	6	7	8	9	10	11

SUNDAY

Goal	12	1	2	3	4	5	6	7	8	9	10	11	12	1	2	3	4	5	6	7	8	9	10	11
Actual	12	1	2	3	4	5	6	7	8	9	10	11	12	1	2	3	4	5	6	7	8	9	10	11

21 DAY KETO *Challenge*

It takes just 21 days to create a healthy routine that will last a lifetime!

START DATE	END DATE

1	2	3	4	5
6	7	8	9	10
11	12	13	14	15
16	17	18	19	20

21	NOTES

Keto Grocery Inventory

DATE: _____

QTY	PRODUCE

QTY	MEAT & FISH

QTY	FROZEN FOODS

QTY	DAIRY

QTY	PANTRY

QTY	OTHER/MISC.

WEIGHT LOSS *Journal*

MONDAY

WEEK OF:

DATE	WEIGHT LOSS ACTION PLAN

TUESDAY

WEDNESDAY

THURSDAY

FRIDAY

SATURDAY

NOTES

SUNDAY

WEIGHT LOSS *Tracker*

MONTHLY GOAL

DATE:

	BUST				
	WAIST				
	HIPS				
	BICEP				
	THIGH				
	CALF				
	WEIGHT				

TOTAL WEIGHT LOSS >>

MONTHLY PROGRESS *Tracker*

JAN	FEB	MAR	APR	MAY	JUN	JUL	AUG	SEP	OCT	NOV	DEC

MON	TUE	WED	THU	FRI	SAT	SUN

WEIGHT LOSS MILESTONE TRACKER

CHEAT DAY TRACKER

WEEKLY DIET SUCCESS TRACKER & NOTES

MY WEIGHT LOSS *Routine*

CREATING A ROUTINE FOR SUCCESS

WEIGHT LOSS SUCCESS: HABIT & ROUTINE TRACKER	
DRINK LOTS OF WATER TODAY	**TRACK TOTAL CARB INTAKE**

COMPLETE TOP 3 GOALS OF THE DAY

1
2
3

PLAN MY MEALS FOR THE DAY:

BREAKFAST	LUNCH	DINNER

DAILY TRACKER & TO DO LIST	ACCOMPLISHMENTS

NOTES

MY KETO *Routine*

Morning	My Weight Loss Routine	m t w t f s s

Mid Day	My Weight Loss Routine	m t w t f s s

Evening	My Weight Loss Routine	m t w t f s s

Night	My Weight Loss Routine	m t w t f s s

WEEKLY *Fasting Tracker*

Week Of: _____

MONDAY

Goal	12	1	2	3	4	5	6	7	8	9	10	11	12	1	2	3	4	5	6	7	8	9	10	11
Actual	12	1	2	3	4	5	6	7	8	9	10	11	12	1	2	3	4	5	6	7	8	9	10	11

TUESDAY

Goal	12	1	2	3	4	5	6	7	8	9	10	11	12	1	2	3	4	5	6	7	8	9	10	11
Actual	12	1	2	3	4	5	6	7	8	9	10	11	12	1	2	3	4	5	6	7	8	9	10	11

WEDNESDAY

Goal	12	1	2	3	4	5	6	7	8	9	10	11	12	1	2	3	4	5	6	7	8	9	10	11
Actual	12	1	2	3	4	5	6	7	8	9	10	11	12	1	2	3	4	5	6	7	8	9	10	11

THURSDAY

Goal	12	1	2	3	4	5	6	7	8	9	10	11	12	1	2	3	4	5	6	7	8	9	10	11
Actual	12	1	2	3	4	5	6	7	8	9	10	11	12	1	2	3	4	5	6	7	8	9	10	11

FRIDAY

Goal	12	1	2	3	4	5	6	7	8	9	10	11	12	1	2	3	4	5	6	7	8	9	10	11
Actual	12	1	2	3	4	5	6	7	8	9	10	11	12	1	2	3	4	5	6	7	8	9	10	11

SATURDAY

Goal	12	1	2	3	4	5	6	7	8	9	10	11	12	1	2	3	4	5	6	7	8	9	10	11
Actual	12	1	2	3	4	5	6	7	8	9	10	11	12	1	2	3	4	5	6	7	8	9	10	11

SUNDAY

Goal	12	1	2	3	4	5	6	7	8	9	10	11	12	1	2	3	4	5	6	7	8	9	10	11
Actual	12	1	2	3	4	5	6	7	8	9	10	11	12	1	2	3	4	5	6	7	8	9	10	11

WEEK OF:

KETO *Meal* LOG BOOK

	BREAKFAST	LUNCH	DINNER	SNACKS
MONDAY				
TUESDAY				
WEDNESDAY				
THURSDAY				
FRIDAY				
SATURDAY				
SUNDAY				

MY PROGRESS *Tracker*

SLEEP TRACKER:

DATE _____

 RISE: | BEDTIME: | SLEEP (HRS):

NOTES FOR THE DAY

IN A STATE OF KETOSIS?

YES   NO   UNSURE

WATER INTAKE TRACKER

EXERCISE / WORKOUT ROUTINE

DAILY ENERGY LEVEL		
HIGH	**MEDIUM**	**LOW**

BREAKFAST

FAT: CARBS: PROTEIN: CALORIES:

LUNCH

FAT: CARBS: PROTEIN: CALORIES:

DINNER

FAT: CARBS: PROTEIN: CALORIES:

SNACKS

FAT: CARBS: PROTEIN: CALORIES:

TOP 6 PRIORITIES OF THE DAY

END OF THE DAY TOTAL OVERVIEW

CARBS   FAT   PROTEIN   CALORIES

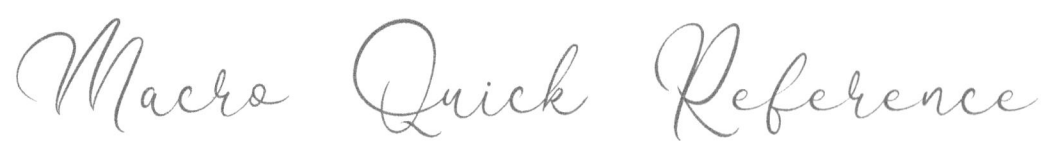

MACRO TRACKER

QTY	TYPE	PROTEIN	FAT	CARBS	CALS	NOTES

INTERMITTENT *Fasting Log*

WEEK OF:

	START TIME	END TIME	TOTAL FAST HRS
M	:	:	:
T	:	:	:
W	:	:	:
T	:	:	:
F	:	:	:
S	:	:	:
S	:	:	:

WEEK OF:

	START TIME	END TIME	TOTAL FAST HRS
M	:	:	:
T	:	:	:
W	:	:	:
T	:	:	:
F	:	:	:
S	:	:	:
S	:	:	:

WEEK OF:

	START TIME	END TIME	TOTAL FAST HRS
M	:	:	:
T	:	:	:
W	:	:	:
T	:	:	:
F	:	:	:
S	:	:	:
S	:	:	:

WEEK OF:

	START TIME	END TIME	TOTAL FAST HRS
M	:	:	:
T	:	:	:
W	:	:	:
T	:	:	:
F	:	:	:
S	:	:	:
S	:	:	:

WEEK OF:

	START TIME	END TIME	TOTAL FAST HRS
M	:	:	:
T	:	:	:
W	:	:	:
T	:	:	:
F	:	:	:
S	:	:	:
S	:	:	:

WEEK OF:

	START TIME	END TIME	TOTAL FAST HRS
M	:	:	:
T	:	:	:
W	:	:	:
T	:	:	:
F	:	:	:
S	:	:	:
S	:	:	:

MILESTONES & ACCOMPLISHMENTS

NOTES & REFLECTIONS

GOALS & *Accomplishments*

Month | JAN FEB MAR APR MAY JUN JUL AUG SEP OCT NOV DEC

THIS MONTH'S **GOALS**

ACTION PLAN

M T W T F S S

WEEKLY GOALS

M

T

W

T

F

S

S

NOTES:

THOUGHTS

MEALS:	BREAKFAST	LUNCH	DINNER	SNACKS
M				
T				
W				
T				
F				
S				
S				

Low Carb Shopping List

FRESH PRODUCE

MEAT AND SEAFOOD

DAIRY PRODUCTS

PANTRY ITEMS

FROZEN / OTHER

Keto Friendly Foods

KETO FRIENDLY FOODS	NET CARBS	PROTEINS	FAT

FOODS TO EAT IN MODERATION	NET CARBS	PROTEINS	FAT

STAYING *On Track*

MY WEIGHT LOSS DIARY:

WATER TRACKER

LOW CARB SNACKS

NOTES & REMINDERS

DOODLE MY MOOD

BREAKFAST IDEAS

LUNCH IDEAS

DINNER IDEAS

STAYING *On Track*

MY WEIGHT LOSS DIARY:

WATER TRACKER

NOTES & REMINDERS

DOODLE MY MOOD

LOW CARB SNACKS

BREAKFAST IDEAS

LUNCH IDEAS

DINNER IDEAS

STAYING *On Track*

MY WEIGHT LOSS DIARY:

_____

_____

_____

_____

WATER TRACKER

NOTES & REMINDERS

DOODLE MY MOOD

LOW CARB SNACKS

BREAKFAST IDEAS

LUNCH IDEAS

DINNER IDEAS

STAYING *On Track*

MY WEIGHT LOSS DIARY:

WATER TRACKER

LOW CARB SNACKS

NOTES & REMINDERS

DOODLE MY MOOD

BREAKFAST IDEAS

LUNCH IDEAS

DINNER IDEAS

STAYING *On Track*

MY WEIGHT LOSS DIARY:

_____
_____
_____
_____

WATER TRACKER

LOW CARB SNACKS

NOTES & REMINDERS

DOODLE MY MOOD

BREAKFAST IDEAS

LUNCH IDEAS

DINNER IDEAS

STAYING *On Track*

MY WEIGHT LOSS DIARY:

WATER TRACKER

LOW CARB SNACKS

NOTES & REMINDERS

DOODLE MY MOOD

BREAKFAST IDEAS

LUNCH IDEAS

DINNER IDEAS

STAYING *On Track*

MY WEIGHT LOSS DIARY:

_____

_____

_____

_____

WATER TRACKER

◊ ◊ ◊ ◊ ◊ ◊ ◊

LOW CARB SNACKS

NOTES & REMINDERS

_____

_____

_____

_____

_____

_____

_____

_____

DOODLE MY MOOD

BREAKFAST IDEAS

LUNCH IDEAS

DINNER IDEAS

MEAL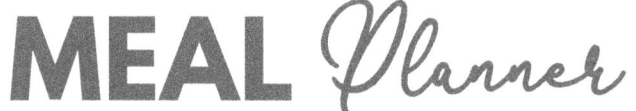

WEEK OF

GROCERY LIST

MON

TUES

WED

THUR

FRI

SAT

SUN

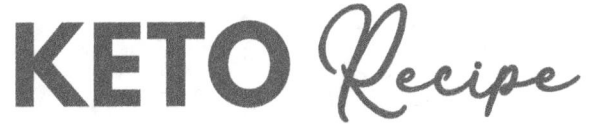

KETO *Recipe*

RECIPE NAME:

	Keto	Low Carb	Paleo	Vegetarian	Vegan	Dairy Free	Gluten Free
	☐	☐	☐	☐	☐	☐	☐

QTY	INGREDIENTS	RECIPE INSTRUCTIONS

NOTES & RECIPE REVIEW

Serves	
Prep Time	
Cook Time	
Tools	
Temp	

Total	Carbs	Fat	Protein	Cals

DAILY FOOD *Tracker*

FOOD TRACKER

MEAL/SNACK	NET CARBS	FAT	CAL	PROTEIN
DAILY GOAL:				
TOTAL:				

FITNESS TRACKER

Type		Notes
Time		
Avg HR		
Max HR		
Reps		
Cals		

DAILY OVERVIEW

Sleep		Notes		On Track
Water Intake				
Steps Taken				
Active Mins				Goal Met
Active Hours				
Cals Burned				

DAILY FOOD *Tracker*

FOOD TRACKER

MEAL/SNACK	NET CARBS	FAT	CAL	PROTEIN
DAILY GOAL:				
TOTAL:				

NOTES & MEAL IDEAS

FITNESS TRACKER

		Notes
Type		
Time		
Avg HR		
Max HR		
Reps		
Cals		

DAILY OVERVIEW

		Notes		On Track
Sleep				
Water Intake				
Steps Taken				
Active Mins				Goal Met
Active Hours				
Cals Burned				

DAILY FOOD *Tracker*

FOOD TRACKER

MEAL/SNACK	NET CARBS	FAT	CAL	PROTEIN

DAILY GOAL:

TOTAL:

NOTES & MEAL IDEAS

FITNESS TRACKER

Type		Notes
Time		
Avg HR		
Max HR		
Reps		
Cals		

DAILY OVERVIEW

Sleep		Notes
Water Intake		
Steps Taken		
Active Mins		
Active Hours		
Cals Burned		

On Track

Goal Met

DAILY FOOD *Tracker*

FOOD TRACKER

MEAL/SNACK	NET CARBS	FAT	CAL	PROTEIN
DAILY GOAL:				
TOTAL:				

NOTES & MEAL IDEAS

FITNESS TRACKER

Type	
Time	
Avg HR	
Max HR	
Reps	
Cals	

Notes

DAILY OVERVIEW

Sleep	
Water Intake	
Steps Taken	
Active Mins	
Active Hours	
Cals Burned	

Notes

On Track

Goal Met

DAILY FOOD *Tracker*

FOOD TRACKER

MEAL/SNACK	NET CARBS	FAT	CAL	PROTEIN
DAILY GOAL:				
TOTAL:				

NOTES & MEAL IDEAS

FITNESS TRACKER

Type		Notes
Time		
Avg HR		
Max HR		
Reps		
Cals		

DAILY OVERVIEW

Sleep		Notes
Water Intake		
Steps Taken		
Active Mins		
Active Hours		
Cals Burned		

On Track

Goal Met

DAILY FOOD *Tracker*

FOOD TRACKER

MEAL/SNACK	NET CARBS	FAT	CAL	PROTEIN
DAILY GOAL:				
TOTAL:				

NOTES & MEAL IDEAS

FITNESS TRACKER

		Notes
Type		
Time		
Avg HR		
Max HR		
Reps		
Cals		

DAILY OVERVIEW

		Notes		
Sleep			On Track	
Water Intake				
Steps Taken				
Active Mins			Goal Met	
Active Hours				
Cals Burned				

DAILY FOOD *Tracker*

FOOD TRACKER

MEAL/SNACK	NET CARBS	FAT	CAL	PROTEIN
DAILY GOAL:				
TOTAL:				

NOTES & MEAL IDEAS

FITNESS TRACKER

		Notes
Type		
Time		
Avg HR		
Max HR		
Reps		
Cals		

DAILY OVERVIEW

		Notes			
Sleep				On Track	
Water Intake					
Steps Taken					
Active Mins				Goal Met	
Active Hours					
Cals Burned					

KETO GO TO *Meals*

BREAKFAST	LUNCH	DINNER	SNACKS
BREAKFAST	LUNCH	DINNER	SNACKS
BREAKFAST	LUNCH	DINNER	SNACKS
BREAKFAST	LUNCH	DINNER	SNACKS
BREAKFAST	LUNCH	DINNER	SNACKS
BREAKFAST	LUNCH	DINNER	SNACKS
BREAKFAST	LUNCH	DINNER	SNACKS

12 WEEK *Keto Meal Tracker*

MONTH	JAN	FEB	MAR	APR	MAY	JUN	JUL	AUG	SEP	OCT	NOV	DEC
WEEK	01	02	03	04	05	06	07	08	09	10	11	12

	BREAKFAST	LUNCH	DINNER	SNACKS
M				
T				
W				
T				
F				
S				
S				

GROCERY SHOPPING LIST / RECIPE INGREDIENTS

Weekly Meal Planner

Week of: _____

	Breakfast	Lunch	Dinner	Snack	Other
Monday	TOTAL Carbs Fat Protein Cals	TOTAL Carbs Fat Protein Cals	TOTAL Carbs Fat Protein Cals	TOTAL Carbs Fat Protein Cals	TOTAL Carbs Fat Protein Cals
Tuesday	TOTAL Carbs Fat Protein Cals	TOTAL Carbs Fat Protein Cals	TOTAL Carbs Fat Protein Cals	TOTAL Carbs Fat Protein Cals	TOTAL Carbs Fat Protein Cals
Wednesday	TOTAL Carbs Fat Protein Cals	TOTAL Carbs Fat Protein Cals	TOTAL Carbs Fat Protein Cals	TOTAL Carbs Fat Protein Cals	TOTAL Carbs Fat Protein Cals
Thursday	TOTAL Carbs Fat Protein Cals	TOTAL Carbs Fat Protein Cals	TOTAL Carbs Fat Protein Cals	TOTAL Carbs Fat Protein Cals	TOTAL Carbs Fat Protein Cals
Friday	TOTAL Carbs Fat Protein Cals	TOTAL Carbs Fat Protein Cals	TOTAL Carbs Fat Protein Cals	TOTAL Carbs Fat Protein Cals	TOTAL Carbs Fat Protein Cals
Saturday	TOTAL Carbs Fat Protein Cals	TOTAL Carbs Fat Protein Cals	TOTAL Carbs Fat Protein Cals	TOTAL Carbs Fat Protein Cals	TOTAL Carbs Fat Protein Cals
Sunday	TOTAL Carbs Fat Protein Cals	TOTAL Carbs Fat Protein Cals	TOTAL Carbs Fat Protein Cals	TOTAL Carbs Fat Protein Cals	TOTAL Carbs Fat Protein Cals

WEIGHT LOSS *Journal*

MONDAY

TUESDAY

WEDNESDAY

THURSDAY

FRIDAY

SATURDAY

SUNDAY

WEEK OF:

DATE	WEIGHT LOSS ACTION PLAN

NOTES

MY WEIGHT LOSS *Routine*

CREATING A ROUTINE FOR SUCCESS

WEIGHT LOSS SUCCESS: HABIT & ROUTINE TRACKER	
DRINK LOTS OF WATER TODAY	**TRACK TOTAL CARB INTAKE**

COMPLETE TOP 3 GOALS OF THE DAY

1
2
3

PLAN MY MEALS FOR THE DAY:

BREAKFAST	LUNCH	DINNER

DAILY TRACKER & TO DO LIST	ACCOMPLISHMENTS

NOTES

MY KETO *Routine*

Morning   *My Weight Loss Routine*   m t w t f s s

Mid Day   *My Weight Loss Routine*   m t w t f s s

Evening   *My Weight Loss Routine*   m t w t f s s

Night   *My Weight Loss Routine*   m t w t f s s

WEEKLY *Fasting Tracker*

Week Of: _____

MONDAY

Goal	12	1	2	3	4	5	6	7	8	9	10	11	12	1	2	3	4	5	6	7	8	9	10	11
Actual	12	1	2	3	4	5	6	7	8	9	10	11	12	1	2	3	4	5	6	7	8	9	10	11

TUESDAY

Goal	12	1	2	3	4	5	6	7	8	9	10	11	12	1	2	3	4	5	6	7	8	9	10	11
Actual	12	1	2	3	4	5	6	7	8	9	10	11	12	1	2	3	4	5	6	7	8	9	10	11

WEDNESDAY

Goal	12	1	2	3	4	5	6	7	8	9	10	11	12	1	2	3	4	5	6	7	8	9	10	11
Actual	12	1	2	3	4	5	6	7	8	9	10	11	12	1	2	3	4	5	6	7	8	9	10	11

THURSDAY

Goal	12	1	2	3	4	5	6	7	8	9	10	11	12	1	2	3	4	5	6	7	8	9	10	11
Actual	12	1	2	3	4	5	6	7	8	9	10	11	12	1	2	3	4	5	6	7	8	9	10	11

FRIDAY

Goal	12	1	2	3	4	5	6	7	8	9	10	11	12	1	2	3	4	5	6	7	8	9	10	11
Actual	12	1	2	3	4	5	6	7	8	9	10	11	12	1	2	3	4	5	6	7	8	9	10	11

SATURDAY

Goal	12	1	2	3	4	5	6	7	8	9	10	11	12	1	2	3	4	5	6	7	8	9	10	11
Actual	12	1	2	3	4	5	6	7	8	9	10	11	12	1	2	3	4	5	6	7	8	9	10	11

SUNDAY

Goal	12	1	2	3	4	5	6	7	8	9	10	11	12	1	2	3	4	5	6	7	8	9	10	11
Actual	12	1	2	3	4	5	6	7	8	9	10	11	12	1	2	3	4	5	6	7	8	9	10	11

WEEK OF:

KETO *Meal* LOG BOOK

	BREAKFAST	LUNCH	DINNER	SNACKS
MONDAY				
TUESDAY				
WEDNESDAY				
THURSDAY				
FRIDAY				
SATURDAY				
SUNDAY				

MY PROGRESS *Tracker*

SLEEP TRACKER:

DATE _____

RISE: _____   BEDTIME: _____   SLEEP (HRS): _____

NOTES FOR THE DAY

_____

_____

_____

IN A STATE OF KETOSIS?

YES   NO   UNSURE

WATER INTAKE TRACKER

EXERCISE / WORKOUT ROUTINE

DAILY ENERGY LEVEL		
HIGH	**MEDIUM**	**LOW**

BREAKFAST

FAT: CARBS: PROTEIN: CALORIES:

LUNCH

FAT: CARBS: PROTEIN: CALORIES:

DINNER

FAT: CARBS: PROTEIN: CALORIES:

SNACKS

FAT: CARBS: PROTEIN: CALORIES:

TOP 6 PRIORITIES OF THE DAY

END OF THE DAY TOTAL OVERVIEW

CARBS	FAT	PROTEIN	CALORIES

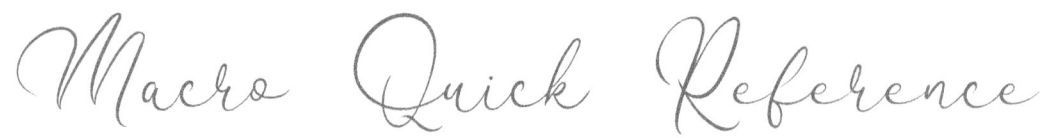

MACRO TRACKER

QTY	TYPE	PROTEIN	FAT	CARBS	CALS	NOTES

INTERMITTENT *Fasting Log*

WEEK OF:

	START TIME	END TIME	TOTAL FAST HRS
M	:	:	:
T	:	:	:
W	:	:	:
T	:	:	:
F	:	:	:
S	:	:	:
S	:	:	:

WEEK OF:

	START TIME	END TIME	TOTAL FAST HRS
M	:	:	:
T	:	:	:
W	:	:	:
T	:	:	:
F	:	:	:
S	:	:	:
S	:	:	:

WEEK OF:

	START TIME	END TIME	TOTAL FAST HRS
M	:	:	:
T	:	:	:
W	:	:	:
T	:	:	:
F	:	:	:
S	:	:	:
S	:	:	:

WEEK OF:

	START TIME	END TIME	TOTAL FAST HRS
M	:	:	:
T	:	:	:
W	:	:	:
T	:	:	:
F	:	:	:
S	:	:	:
S	:	:	:

WEEK OF:

	START TIME	END TIME	TOTAL FAST HRS
M	:	:	:
T	:	:	:
W	:	:	:
T	:	:	:
F	:	:	:
S	:	:	:
S	:	:	:

WEEK OF:

	START TIME	END TIME	TOTAL FAST HRS
M	:	:	:
T	:	:	:
W	:	:	:
T	:	:	:
F	:	:	:
S	:	:	:
S	:	:	:

MILESTONES & ACCOMPLISHMENTS

NOTES & REFLECTIONS

GOALS & *Accomplishments*

Month | JAN FEB MAR APR MAY JUN JUL AUG SEP OCT NOV DEC

THIS MONTH'S **GOALS**

ACTION PLAN

M T W T F S S

☐☐☐☐☐☐☐
☐☐☐☐☐☐☐
☐☐☐☐☐☐☐
☐☐☐☐☐☐☐
☐☐☐☐☐☐☐

NOTES:

WEEKLY GOALS

M

T

W

T

F

S

S

THOUGHTS

MEALS:	BREAKFAST	LUNCH	DINNER	SNACKS
M				
T				
W				
T				
F				
S				
S				

Low Carb Shopping List

FRESH PRODUCE

MEAT AND SEAFOOD

DAIRY PRODUCTS

PANTRY ITEMS

FROZEN / OTHER

Keto Friendly Foods

KETO FRIENDLY FOODS	NET CARBS	PROTEINS	FAT

FOODS TO EAT IN MODERATION	NET CARBS	PROTEINS	FAT

STAYING *On Track*

MY WEIGHT LOSS DIARY:

_____

_____

_____

_____

WATER TRACKER

◇ ◇ ◇ ◇ ◇ ◇ ◇ ◇

LOW CARB SNACKS

NOTES & REMINDERS

_____

_____

_____

_____

_____

_____

_____

_____

DOODLE MY MOOD

BREAKFAST IDEAS

LUNCH IDEAS

DINNER IDEAS

STAYING *On Track*

MY WEIGHT LOSS DIARY:

WATER TRACKER

NOTES & REMINDERS

DOODLE MY MOOD

LOW CARB SNACKS

BREAKFAST IDEAS

LUNCH IDEAS

DINNER IDEAS

STAYING *On Track*

MY WEIGHT LOSS DIARY:

_____

_____

_____

_____

WATER TRACKER

NOTES & REMINDERS

DOODLE MY MOOD

LOW CARB SNACKS

BREAKFAST IDEAS

LUNCH IDEAS

DINNER IDEAS

STAYING *On Track*

MY WEIGHT LOSS DIARY:

WATER TRACKER

○ ○ ○ ○ ○ ○ ○ ○

NOTES & REMINDERS

DOODLE MY MOOD

LOW CARB SNACKS

BREAKFAST IDEAS

LUNCH IDEAS

DINNER IDEAS

STAYING *On Track*

MY WEIGHT LOSS DIARY:

_____

_____

_____

_____

WATER TRACKER

LOW CARB SNACKS

NOTES & REMINDERS

DOODLE MY MOOD

BREAKFAST IDEAS

LUNCH IDEAS

DINNER IDEAS

STAYING *On Track*

MY WEIGHT LOSS DIARY:

WATER TRACKER

NOTES & REMINDERS

DOODLE MY MOOD

LOW CARB SNACKS

BREAKFAST IDEAS

LUNCH IDEAS

DINNER IDEAS

STAYING *On Track*

MY WEIGHT LOSS DIARY:

_____

_____

_____

_____

WATER TRACKER

◊ ◊ ◊ ◊ ◊ ◊ ◊

LOW CARB SNACKS

NOTES & REMINDERS

_____

_____

_____

_____

_____

_____

_____

_____

_____

_____

DOODLE MY MOOD

BREAKFAST IDEAS

LUNCH IDEAS

DINNER IDEAS

MEAL *Planner*

WEEK OF

GROCERY LIST

- [ ]
- [ ]
- [ ]
- [ ]
- [ ]
- [ ]
- [ ]
- [ ]
- [ ]
- [ ]
- [ ]
- [ ]
- [ ]
- [ ]
- [ ]
- [ ]

MON

TUES

WED

THUR

FRI

SAT

SUN

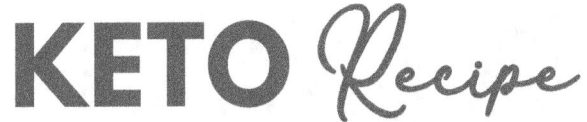

KETO *Recipe*

RECIPE NAME:

	Keto	Low Carb	Paleo	Vegetarian	Vegan	Dairy Free	Gluten Free
	☐	☐	☐	☐	☐	☐	☐

QTY	INGREDIENTS

RECIPE INSTRUCTIONS

NOTES & RECIPE REVIEW

Serves	
Prep Time	
Cook Time	
Tools	
Temp	

Total	Carbs	Fat	Protein	Cals

DAILY FOOD *Tracker*

FOOD TRACKER

MEAL/SNACK	NET CARBS	FAT	CAL	PROTEIN
DAILY GOAL:				
TOTAL:				

NOTES & MEAL IDEAS

FITNESS TRACKER

		Notes
Type		
Time		
Avg HR		
Max HR		
Reps		
Cals		

DAILY OVERVIEW

		Notes		
Sleep			On Track	
Water Intake				
Steps Taken				
Active Mins			Goal Met	
Active Hours				
Cals Burned				

DAILY FOOD *Tracker*

FOOD TRACKER

MEAL/SNACK	NET CARBS	FAT	CAL	PROTEIN
DAILY GOAL:				
TOTAL:				

NOTES & MEAL IDEAS

FITNESS TRACKER

Type		Notes
Time		
Avg HR		
Max HR		
Reps		
Cals		

DAILY OVERVIEW

Sleep		Notes		On Track
Water Intake				
Steps Taken				
Active Mins				Goal Met
Active Hours				
Cals Burned				

DAILY FOOD *Tracker*

FOOD TRACKER

MEAL/SNACK	NET CARBS	FAT	CAL	PROTEIN
DAILY GOAL:				
TOTAL:				

NOTES & MEAL IDEAS

FITNESS TRACKER

		Notes
Type		
Time		
Avg HR		
Max HR		
Reps		
Cals		

DAILY OVERVIEW

		Notes		
Sleep			On Track	
Water Intake				
Steps Taken				
Active Mins			Goal Met	
Active Hours				
Cals Burned				

DAILY FOOD *Tracker*

FOOD TRACKER

MEAL/SNACK	NET CARBS	FAT	CAL	PROTEIN
DAILY GOAL:				
TOTAL:				

NOTES & MEAL IDEAS

FITNESS TRACKER

Type		Notes
Time		
Avg HR		
Max HR		
Reps		
Cals		

DAILY OVERVIEW

Sleep		Notes		On Track
Water Intake				
Steps Taken				
Active Mins				Goal Met
Active Hours				
Cals Burned				

DAILY FOOD *Tracker*

FOOD TRACKER

MEAL/SNACK	NET CARBS	FAT	CAL	PROTEIN
DAILY GOAL:				
TOTAL:				

NOTES & MEAL IDEAS

FITNESS TRACKER

		Notes
Type		
Time		
Avg HR		
Max HR		
Reps		
Cals		

DAILY OVERVIEW

		Notes		
Sleep				On Track
Water Intake				
Steps Taken				
Active Mins				Goal Met
Active Hours				
Cals Burned				

DAILY FOOD *Tracker*

FOOD TRACKER

MEAL/SNACK	NET CARBS	FAT	CAL	PROTEIN
DAILY GOAL:				
TOTAL:				

NOTES & MEAL IDEAS

FITNESS TRACKER

Type		Notes
Time		
Avg HR		
Max HR		
Reps		
Cals		

DAILY OVERVIEW

Sleep		Notes		On Track
Water Intake				
Steps Taken				
Active Mins				Goal Met
Active Hours				
Cals Burned				

DAILY FOOD *Tracker*

FOOD TRACKER

MEAL/SNACK	NET CARBS	FAT	CAL	PROTEIN
DAILY GOAL:				
TOTAL:				

NOTES & MEAL IDEAS

FITNESS TRACKER

		Notes
Type		
Time		
Avg HR		
Max HR		
Reps		
Cals		

DAILY OVERVIEW

		Notes		On Track
Sleep				
Water Intake				
Steps Taken				
Active Mins				Goal Met
Active Hours				
Cals Burned				

KETO GO TO *Meals*

BREAKFAST	LUNCH	DINNER	SNACKS
BREAKFAST	LUNCH	DINNER	SNACKS
BREAKFAST	LUNCH	DINNER	SNACKS
BREAKFAST	LUNCH	DINNER	SNACKS
BREAKFAST	LUNCH	DINNER	SNACKS
BREAKFAST	LUNCH	DINNER	SNACKS
BREAKFAST	LUNCH	DINNER	SNACKS

12 WEEK *Keto Meal Tracker*

12 Week Keto Challenge

MONTH	JAN	FEB	MAR	APR	MAY	JUN	JUL	AUG	SEP	OCT	NOV	DEC
WEEK	01	02	03	04	05	06	07	08	09	10	11	12

	BREAKFAST	LUNCH	DINNER	SNACKS
M				
T				
W				
T				
F				
S				
S				

GROCERY SHOPPING LIST / RECIPE INGREDIENTS

Weekly Meal Planner

Week of: _____

	Breakfast	Lunch	Dinner	Snack	Other
Monday	TOTAL Carbs Fat Protein Cals	TOTAL Carbs Fat Protein Cals	TOTAL Carbs Fat Protein Cals	TOTAL Carbs Fat Protein Cals	TOTAL Carbs Fat Protein Cals
Tuesday	TOTAL Carbs Fat Protein Cals	TOTAL Carbs Fat Protein Cals	TOTAL Carbs Fat Protein Cals	TOTAL Carbs Fat Protein Cals	TOTAL Carbs Fat Protein Cals
Wednesday	TOTAL Carbs Fat Protein Cals	TOTAL Carbs Fat Protein Cals	TOTAL Carbs Fat Protein Cals	TOTAL Carbs Fat Protein Cals	TOTAL Carbs Fat Protein Cals
Thursday	TOTAL Carbs Fat Protein Cals	TOTAL Carbs Fat Protein Cals	TOTAL Carbs Fat Protein Cals	TOTAL Carbs Fat Protein Cals	TOTAL Carbs Fat Protein Cals
Friday	TOTAL Carbs Fat Protein Cals	TOTAL Carbs Fat Protein Cals	TOTAL Carbs Fat Protein Cals	TOTAL Carbs Fat Protein Cals	TOTAL Carbs Fat Protein Cals
Saturday	TOTAL Carbs Fat Protein Cals	TOTAL Carbs Fat Protein Cals	TOTAL Carbs Fat Protein Cals	TOTAL Carbs Fat Protein Cals	TOTAL Carbs Fat Protein Cals
Sunday	TOTAL Carbs Fat Protein Cals	TOTAL Carbs Fat Protein Cals	TOTAL Carbs Fat Protein Cals	TOTAL Carbs Fat Protein Cals	TOTAL Carbs Fat Protein Cals

WEIGHT LOSS *Journal*

MONDAY

WEEK OF:

DATE	WEIGHT LOSS ACTION PLAN

TUESDAY

WEDNESDAY

THURSDAY

FRIDAY

SATURDAY

NOTES

SUNDAY

MY WEIGHT LOSS *Routine*

CREATING A ROUTINE FOR SUCCESS

WEIGHT LOSS SUCCESS: HABIT & ROUTINE TRACKER	
DRINK LOTS OF WATER TODAY	TRACK TOTAL CARB INTAKE

COMPLETE TOP 3 GOALS OF THE DAY

1

2

3

PLAN MY MEALS FOR THE DAY:

BREAKFAST	LUNCH	DINNER

DAILY TRACKER & TO DO LIST	ACCOMPLISHMENTS

NOTES

WEEKLY *Fasting Tracker*

Week Of: _____

MONDAY

Goal	12	1	2	3	4	5	6	7	8	9	10	11	12	1	2	3	4	5	6	7	8	9	10	11
Actual	12	1	2	3	4	5	6	7	8	9	10	11	12	1	2	3	4	5	6	7	8	9	10	11

TUESDAY

Goal	12	1	2	3	4	5	6	7	8	9	10	11	12	1	2	3	4	5	6	7	8	9	10	11
Actual	12	1	2	3	4	5	6	7	8	9	10	11	12	1	2	3	4	5	6	7	8	9	10	11

WEDNESDAY

Goal	12	1	2	3	4	5	6	7	8	9	10	11	12	1	2	3	4	5	6	7	8	9	10	11
Actual	12	1	2	3	4	5	6	7	8	9	10	11	12	1	2	3	4	5	6	7	8	9	10	11

THURSDAY

Goal	12	1	2	3	4	5	6	7	8	9	10	11	12	1	2	3	4	5	6	7	8	9	10	11
Actual	12	1	2	3	4	5	6	7	8	9	10	11	12	1	2	3	4	5	6	7	8	9	10	11

FRIDAY

Goal	12	1	2	3	4	5	6	7	8	9	10	11	12	1	2	3	4	5	6	7	8	9	10	11
Actual	12	1	2	3	4	5	6	7	8	9	10	11	12	1	2	3	4	5	6	7	8	9	10	11

SATURDAY

Goal	12	1	2	3	4	5	6	7	8	9	10	11	12	1	2	3	4	5	6	7	8	9	10	11
Actual	12	1	2	3	4	5	6	7	8	9	10	11	12	1	2	3	4	5	6	7	8	9	10	11

SUNDAY

Goal	12	1	2	3	4	5	6	7	8	9	10	11	12	1	2	3	4	5	6	7	8	9	10	11
Actual	12	1	2	3	4	5	6	7	8	9	10	11	12	1	2	3	4	5	6	7	8	9	10	11

WEEKLY *Progress*

Monday

Tuesday

Wednesday

Thursday

Friday

Saturday

Sunday

Notes

WEEK OF:

KETO *Meal* LOG BOOK

	BREAKFAST	LUNCH	DINNER	SNACKS
MONDAY				
TUESDAY				
WEDNESDAY				
THURSDAY				
FRIDAY				
SATURDAY				
SUNDAY				

MY PROGRESS *Tracker*

SLEEP TRACKER:

DATE _____

 RISE: | BEDTIME: | SLEEP (HRS):

NOTES FOR THE DAY

_____

_____

EXERCISE / WORKOUT ROUTINE

TOP 6 PRIORITIES OF THE DAY

IN A STATE OF KETOSIS?

YES   NO   UNSURE

WATER INTAKE TRACKER

DAILY ENERGY LEVEL

HIGH   MEDIUM   LOW

BREAKFAST

FAT: CARBS: PROTEIN: CALORIES:

LUNCH

FAT: CARBS: PROTEIN: CALORIES:

DINNER

FAT: CARBS: PROTEIN: CALORIES:

SNACKS

FAT: CARBS: PROTEIN: CALORIES:

END OF THE DAY TOTAL OVERVIEW

CARBS   FAT   PROTEIN   CALORIES

WEIGHT LOSS *Tracker*

MONTHLY GOAL

DATE:

BUST					
WAIST					
HIPS					
BICEP					
THIGH					
CALF					
WEIGHT					

TOTAL WEIGHT LOSS >>

MONTHLY PROGRESS *Tracker*

JAN	FEB	MAR	APR	MAY	JUN	JUL	AUG	SEP	OCT	NOV	DEC

MON	TUE	WED	THU	FRI	SAT	SUN

WEIGHT LOSS MILESTONE TRACKER

CHEAT DAY TRACKER

WEEKLY DIET SUCCESS TRACKER & NOTES

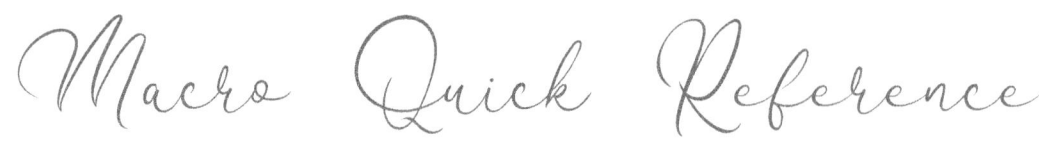

MACRO TRACKER

QTY	TYPE	PROTEIN	FAT	CARBS	CALS	NOTES

INTERMITTENT *Fasting Log*

WEEK OF:

	START TIME	END TIME	TOTAL FAST HRS
M	:	:	:
T	:	:	:
W	:	:	:
T	:	:	:
F	:	:	:
S	:	:	:
S	:	:	:

WEEK OF:

	START TIME	END TIME	TOTAL FAST HRS
M	:	:	:
T	:	:	:
W	:	:	:
T	:	:	:
F	:	:	:
S	:	:	:
S	:	:	:

WEEK OF:

	START TIME	END TIME	TOTAL FAST HRS
M	:	:	:
T	:	:	:
W	:	:	:
T	:	:	:
F	:	:	:
S	:	:	:
S	:	:	:

WEEK OF:

	START TIME	END TIME	TOTAL FAST HRS
M	:	:	:
T	:	:	:
W	:	:	:
T	:	:	:
F	:	:	:
S	:	:	:
S	:	:	:

WEEK OF:

	START TIME	END TIME	TOTAL FAST HRS
M	:	:	:
T	:	:	:
W	:	:	:
T	:	:	:
F	:	:	:
S	:	:	:
S	:	:	:

WEEK OF:

	START TIME	END TIME	TOTAL FAST HRS
M	:	:	:
T	:	:	:
W	:	:	:
T	:	:	:
F	:	:	:
S	:	:	:
S	:	:	:

MILESTONES & ACCOMPLISHMENTS

NOTES & REFLECTIONS

GOALS & *Accomplishments*

THIS MONTH'S **GOALS**

ACTION PLAN

M T W T F S S

WEEKLY GOALS

M
T
W
T
F
S
S

NOTES:

THOUGHTS

MEALS:	BREAKFAST	LUNCH	DINNER	SNACKS
M				
T				
W				
T				
F				
S				
S				

Low Carb Grocery Ideas

FRESH PRODUCE

Asparagus	Cauliflower	Onions
Avocado	Celery	Radishes
Bell Peppers	Cucumber	Salad Mix
Berries	Eggplant	Squash
Broccoli	Fennel	Tomatoes
Brussel Sprouts	Garlic	Bok Choi
Cabbage	Green Beans	Chives
Carrots	Mushrooms	Spinach

MEAT AND SEAFOOD

Bacon	Lamb	Fish
Beef	Pork	Crab
Bison	Rotisserie Chicken	Lobster
Chicken	Sausage	Scallops
Deli meat	Turkey	Shrimp
Ground Beef / Ground Turkey	Oyster	Mussels

DAIRY PRODUCTS

Butter	Eggs	Sour Cream
Cheese	Greek Yogurt, full fat	Ghee
Cream Cheese	Heavy Whipping Cream	Mayo

PANTRY ITEMS

Avocado oil	Tea/Coffee	Moon Cheese
Beef Jerky	Pork Rinds	Low Carb Protein Bars
Bone Broth	Mayonnaise	All Natural Peanut Butter
Tuna, Salmon (canned)	Low Carb Salad Dressing	Stevia
Coconut Butter	Olive oil, extra virgin	Almonds
Coconut Oil	Olives	Spices
Almond Milk	Sweeteners	Almond Flour

FROZEN / OTHER

Low Carb Shopping List

FRESH PRODUCE

MEAT AND SEAFOOD

DAIRY PRODUCTS

PANTRY ITEMS

FROZEN / OTHER

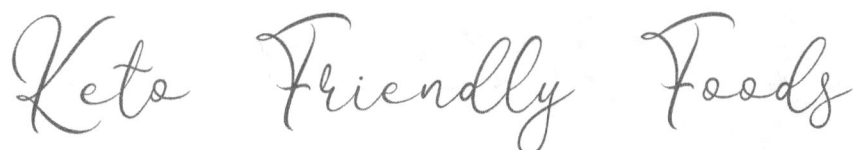

Keto Friendly Foods

KETO FRIENDLY FOODS	NET CARBS	PROTEINS	FAT

FOODS TO EAT IN MODERATION	NET CARBS	PROTEINS	FAT

STAYING *On Track*

MY WEIGHT LOSS DIARY:

WATER TRACKER

LOW CARB SNACKS

NOTES & REMINDERS

DOODLE MY MOOD

BREAKFAST IDEAS

LUNCH IDEAS

DINNER IDEAS

STAYING *On Track*

MY WEIGHT LOSS DIARY:

_____

_____

_____

_____

WATER TRACKER

NOTES & REMINDERS

DOODLE MY MOOD

LOW CARB SNACKS

BREAKFAST IDEAS

LUNCH IDEAS

DINNER IDEAS

STAYING *On Track*

MY WEIGHT LOSS DIARY:

WATER TRACKER

NOTES & REMINDERS

DOODLE MY MOOD

LOW CARB SNACKS

BREAKFAST IDEAS

LUNCH IDEAS

DINNER IDEAS

STAYING *On Track*

MY WEIGHT LOSS DIARY:

_____

_____

_____

_____

WATER TRACKER

NOTES & REMINDERS

DOODLE MY MOOD

LOW CARB SNACKS

BREAKFAST IDEAS

LUNCH IDEAS

DINNER IDEAS

STAYING *On Track*

MY WEIGHT LOSS DIARY:

WATER TRACKER

LOW CARB SNACKS

NOTES & REMINDERS

DOODLE MY MOOD

BREAKFAST IDEAS

LUNCH IDEAS

DINNER IDEAS

STAYING *On Track*

MY WEIGHT LOSS DIARY:

_____

_____

_____

_____

WATER TRACKER

LOW CARB SNACKS

NOTES & REMINDERS

DOODLE MY MOOD

BREAKFAST IDEAS

LUNCH IDEAS

DINNER IDEAS

STAYING *On Track*

MY WEIGHT LOSS DIARY:

WATER TRACKER

LOW CARB SNACKS

NOTES & REMINDERS

DOODLE MY MOOD

BREAKFAST IDEAS

LUNCH IDEAS

DINNER IDEAS

MEAL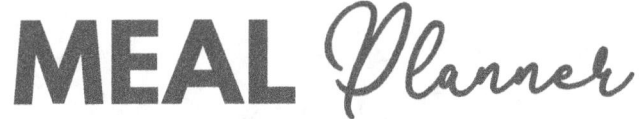

WEEK OF

GROCERY LIST

☐
☐
☐
☐
☐
☐
☐
☐
☐
☐
☐
☐
☐
☐
☐
☐
☐

MON

TUES

WED

THUR

FRI

SAT

SUN

KETO *Recipe*

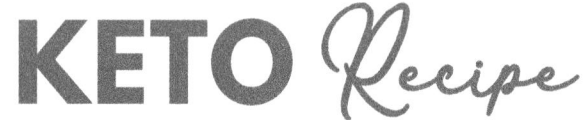

RECIPE NAME:

Keto	Low Carb	Paleo	Vegetarian	Vegan	Dairy Free	Gluten Free
☐	☐	☐	☐	☐	☐	☐

QTY	INGREDIENTS	RECIPE INSTRUCTIONS

NOTES & RECIPE REVIEW

Serves	
Prep Time	
Cook Time	
Tools	
Temp	

Total	Carbs	Fat	Protein	Cals

DAILY FOOD *Tracker*

FOOD TRACKER

MEAL/SNACK	NET CARBS	FAT	CAL	PROTEIN
DAILY GOAL:				
TOTAL:				

NOTES & MEAL IDEAS

FITNESS TRACKER

Type		Notes
Time		
Avg HR		
Max HR		
Reps		
Cals		

DAILY OVERVIEW

Sleep		Notes		On Track
Water Intake				
Steps Taken				
Active Mins				Goal Met
Active Hours				
Cals Burned				

DAILY FOOD *Tracker*

FOOD TRACKER

MEAL/SNACK	NET CARBS	FAT	CAL	PROTEIN
DAILY GOAL:				
TOTAL:				

NOTES & MEAL IDEAS

FITNESS TRACKER

Type		Notes
Time		
Avg HR		
Max HR		
Reps		
Cals		

DAILY OVERVIEW

Sleep		Notes		On Track
Water Intake				
Steps Taken				
Active Mins				Goal Met
Active Hours				
Cals Burned				

DAILY FOOD *Tracker*

FOOD TRACKER

MEAL/SNACK	NET CARBS	FAT	CAL	PROTEIN
DAILY GOAL:				
TOTAL:				

NOTES & MEAL IDEAS

FITNESS TRACKER

Type		Notes
Time		
Avg HR		
Max HR		
Reps		
Cals		

DAILY OVERVIEW

Sleep		Notes		On Track
Water Intake				
Steps Taken				
Active Mins				Goal Met
Active Hours				
Cals Burned				

DAILY FOOD *Tracker*

FOOD TRACKER

MEAL/SNACK	NET CARBS	FAT	CAL	PROTEIN
DAILY GOAL:				
TOTAL:				

NOTES & MEAL IDEAS

FITNESS TRACKER

Type		Notes
Time		
Avg HR		
Max HR		
Reps		
Cals		

DAILY OVERVIEW

Sleep		Notes		On Track
Water Intake				
Steps Taken				☐
Active Mins				Goal Met
Active Hours				
Cals Burned				☐

DAILY FOOD *Tracker*

FOOD TRACKER

MEAL/SNACK	NET CARBS	FAT	CAL	PROTEIN
DAILY GOAL:				
TOTAL:				

NOTES & MEAL IDEAS

FITNESS TRACKER

		Notes
Type		
Time		
Avg HR		
Max HR		
Reps		
Cals		

DAILY OVERVIEW

		Notes		
Sleep			On Track	☐
Water Intake				
Steps Taken				
Active Mins			Goal Met	☐
Active Hours				
Cals Burned				

DAILY FOOD *Tracker*

FOOD TRACKER

MEAL/SNACK	NET CARBS	FAT	CAL	PROTEIN
DAILY GOAL:				
TOTAL:				

NOTES & MEAL IDEAS

FITNESS TRACKER

Type		Notes
Time		
Avg HR		
Max HR		
Reps		
Cals		

DAILY OVERVIEW

Sleep		Notes	On Track
Water Intake			
Steps Taken			
Active Mins			Goal Met
Active Hours			
Cals Burned			

DAILY FOOD *Tracker*

FOOD TRACKER

MEAL/SNACK	NET CARBS	FAT	CAL	PROTEIN
DAILY GOAL:				
TOTAL:				

NOTES & MEAL IDEAS

FITNESS TRACKER

Type		Notes
Time		
Avg HR		
Max HR		
Reps		
Cals		

DAILY OVERVIEW

Sleep		Notes		On Track
Water Intake				
Steps Taken				
Active Mins				Goal Met
Active Hours				
Cals Burned				

KETO GO TO *Meals*

BREAKFAST	LUNCH	DINNER	SNACKS

BREAKFAST	LUNCH	DINNER	SNACKS

BREAKFAST	LUNCH	DINNER	SNACKS

BREAKFAST	LUNCH	DINNER	SNACKS

BREAKFAST	LUNCH	DINNER	SNACKS

BREAKFAST	LUNCH	DINNER	SNACKS

BREAKFAST	LUNCH	DINNER	SNACKS

12 WEEK *Keto Meal Tracker*

12 Week Keto Challenge

MONTH	JAN	FEB	MAR	APR	MAY	JUN	JUL	AUG	SEP	OCT	NOV	DEC
WEEK	01	02	03	04	05	06	07	08	09	10	11	12

	BREAKFAST	LUNCH	DINNER	SNACKS
M				
T				
W				
T				
F				
S				
S				

GROCERY SHOPPING LIST / RECIPE INGREDIENTS

Weekly Meal Planner

Week of: _____

	Breakfast	Lunch	Dinner	Snack	Other
Monday	TOTAL Carbs Fat Protein Cals	TOTAL Carbs Fat Protein Cals	TOTAL Carbs Fat Protein Cals	TOTAL Carbs Fat Protein Cals	TOTAL Carbs Fat Protein Cals
Tuesday	TOTAL Carbs Fat Protein Cals	TOTAL Carbs Fat Protein Cals	TOTAL Carbs Fat Protein Cals	TOTAL Carbs Fat Protein Cals	TOTAL Carbs Fat Protein Cals
Wednesday	TOTAL Carbs Fat Protein Cals	TOTAL Carbs Fat Protein Cals	TOTAL Carbs Fat Protein Cals	TOTAL Carbs Fat Protein Cals	TOTAL Carbs Fat Protein Cals
Thursday	TOTAL Carbs Fat Protein Cals	TOTAL Carbs Fat Protein Cals	TOTAL Carbs Fat Protein Cals	TOTAL Carbs Fat Protein Cals	TOTAL Carbs Fat Protein Cals
Friday	TOTAL Carbs Fat Protein Cals	TOTAL Carbs Fat Protein Cals	TOTAL Carbs Fat Protein Cals	TOTAL Carbs Fat Protein Cals	TOTAL Carbs Fat Protein Cals
Saturday	TOTAL Carbs Fat Protein Cals	TOTAL Carbs Fat Protein Cals	TOTAL Carbs Fat Protein Cals	TOTAL Carbs Fat Protein Cals	TOTAL Carbs Fat Protein Cals
Sunday	TOTAL Carbs Fat Protein Cals	TOTAL Carbs Fat Protein Cals	TOTAL Carbs Fat Protein Cals	TOTAL Carbs Fat Protein Cals	TOTAL Carbs Fat Protein Cals

WEIGHT LOSS *Journal*

MONDAY

TUESDAY

WEDNESDAY

THURSDAY

FRIDAY

SATURDAY

SUNDAY

WEEK OF:

DATE	WEIGHT LOSS ACTION PLAN

NOTES

MY WEIGHT LOSS *Routine*

WEIGHT LOSS SUCCESS: HABIT & ROUTINE TRACKER

DRINK LOTS OF WATER TODAY	TRACK TOTAL CARB INTAKE

COMPLETE TOP 3 GOALS OF THE DAY

1

2

3

PLAN MY MEALS FOR THE DAY:

BREAKFAST	LUNCH	DINNER

DAILY TRACKER & TO DO LIST	ACCOMPLISHMENTS

NOTES

WEEKLY *Fasting Tracker*

Week Of: _____

MONDAY

Goal	12	1	2	3	4	5	6	7	8	9	10	11	12	1	2	3	4	5	6	7	8	9	10	11
Actual	12	1	2	3	4	5	6	7	8	9	10	11	12	1	2	3	4	5	6	7	8	9	10	11

TUESDAY

Goal	12	1	2	3	4	5	6	7	8	9	10	11	12	1	2	3	4	5	6	7	8	9	10	11
Actual	12	1	2	3	4	5	6	7	8	9	10	11	12	1	2	3	4	5	6	7	8	9	10	11

WEDNESDAY

Goal	12	1	2	3	4	5	6	7	8	9	10	11	12	1	2	3	4	5	6	7	8	9	10	11
Actual	12	1	2	3	4	5	6	7	8	9	10	11	12	1	2	3	4	5	6	7	8	9	10	11

THURSDAY

Goal	12	1	2	3	4	5	6	7	8	9	10	11	12	1	2	3	4	5	6	7	8	9	10	11
Actual	12	1	2	3	4	5	6	7	8	9	10	11	12	1	2	3	4	5	6	7	8	9	10	11

FRIDAY

Goal	12	1	2	3	4	5	6	7	8	9	10	11	12	1	2	3	4	5	6	7	8	9	10	11
Actual	12	1	2	3	4	5	6	7	8	9	10	11	12	1	2	3	4	5	6	7	8	9	10	11

SATURDAY

Goal	12	1	2	3	4	5	6	7	8	9	10	11	12	1	2	3	4	5	6	7	8	9	10	11
Actual	12	1	2	3	4	5	6	7	8	9	10	11	12	1	2	3	4	5	6	7	8	9	10	11

SUNDAY

Goal	12	1	2	3	4	5	6	7	8	9	10	11	12	1	2	3	4	5	6	7	8	9	10	11
Actual	12	1	2	3	4	5	6	7	8	9	10	11	12	1	2	3	4	5	6	7	8	9	10	11

WEEKLY *Progress*

WEEK OF : _____

Monday

Tuesday

Wednesday

Thursday

Friday

Saturday

Sunday

Notes

WEEK OF:

KETO *Meal* LOG BOOK

	BREAKFAST	LUNCH	DINNER	SNACKS
MONDAY				
TUESDAY				
WEDNESDAY				
THURSDAY				
FRIDAY				
SATURDAY				
SUNDAY				

MY PROGRESS *Tracker*

SLEEP TRACKER:

DATE

 RISE: BEDTIME: SLEEP (HRS):

NOTES FOR THE DAY

IN A STATE OF KETOSIS?

YES   NO   UNSURE

WATER INTAKE TRACKER

EXERCISE / WORKOUT ROUTINE

DAILY ENERGY LEVEL		
HIGH	**MEDIUM**	**LOW**

BREAKFAST

FAT: CARBS: PROTEIN: CALORIES:

LUNCH

FAT: CARBS: PROTEIN: CALORIES:

DINNER

FAT: CARBS: PROTEIN: CALORIES:

SNACKS

FAT: CARBS: PROTEIN: CALORIES:

TOP 6 PRIORITIES OF THE DAY

END OF THE DAY TOTAL OVERVIEW

CARBS   FAT   PROTEIN   CALORIES

Macro Quick Reference

MACRO TRACKER

QTY	TYPE	PROTEIN	FAT	CARBS	CALS	NOTES

INTERMITTENT *Fasting Log*

WEEK OF:

	START TIME	END TIME	TOTAL FAST HRS
M	:	:	:
T	:	:	:
W	:	:	:
T	:	:	:
F	:	:	:
S	:	:	:
S	:	:	:

WEEK OF:

	START TIME	END TIME	TOTAL FAST HRS
M	:	:	:
T	:	:	:
W	:	:	:
T	:	:	:
F	:	:	:
S	:	:	:
S	:	:	:

WEEK OF:

	START TIME	END TIME	TOTAL FAST HRS
M	:	:	:
T	:	:	:
W	:	:	:
T	:	:	:
F	:	:	:
S	:	:	:
S	:	:	:

WEEK OF:

	START TIME	END TIME	TOTAL FAST HRS
M	:	:	:
T	:	:	:
W	:	:	:
T	:	:	:
F	:	:	:
S	:	:	:
S	:	:	:

WEEK OF:

	START TIME	END TIME	TOTAL FAST HRS
M	:	:	:
T	:	:	:
W	:	:	:
T	:	:	:
F	:	:	:
S	:	:	:
S	:	:	:

WEEK OF:

	START TIME	END TIME	TOTAL FAST HRS
M	:	:	:
T	:	:	:
W	:	:	:
T	:	:	:
F	:	:	:
S	:	:	:
S	:	:	:

MILESTONES & ACCOMPLISHMENTS

NOTES & REFLECTIONS

GOALS & *Accomplishments*

MONTH | JAN FEB MAR APR MAY JUN JUL AUG SEP OCT NOV DEC

THIS MONTH'S **GOALS**

_____   _____

_____   _____

_____   _____

ACTION PLAN

M T W T F S S

_____ ☐ ☐ ☐ ☐ ☐ ☐ ☐

_____ ☐ ☐ ☐ ☐ ☐ ☐ ☐

_____ ☐ ☐ ☐ ☐ ☐ ☐ ☐

_____ ☐ ☐ ☐ ☐ ☐ ☐ ☐

_____ ☐ ☐ ☐ ☐ ☐ ☐ ☐

NOTES:

WEEKLY GOALS

M _____

T _____

W _____

T _____

F _____

S _____

S _____

THOUGHTS

MEALS:	BREAKFAST	LUNCH	DINNER	SNACKS
M				
T				
W				
T				
F				
S				
S				

Low Carb Shopping List

FRESH PRODUCE

MEAT AND SEAFOOD

DAIRY PRODUCTS

PANTRY ITEMS

FROZEN / OTHER

Keto Friendly Foods

KETO FRIENDLY FOODS	NET CARBS	PROTEINS	FAT

FOODS TO EAT IN MODERATION	NET CARBS	PROTEINS	FAT

STAYING *On Track*

MY WEIGHT LOSS DIARY:

WATER TRACKER

LOW CARB SNACKS

NOTES & REMINDERS

DOODLE MY MOOD

BREAKFAST IDEAS

LUNCH IDEAS

DINNER IDEAS

STAYING *On Track*

MY WEIGHT LOSS DIARY:

_____

_____

_____

_____

WATER TRACKER

LOW CARB SNACKS

NOTES & REMINDERS

DOODLE MY MOOD

BREAKFAST IDEAS

LUNCH IDEAS

DINNER IDEAS

STAYING *On Track*

MY WEIGHT LOSS DIARY:

_____

_____

_____

_____

WATER TRACKER

LOW CARB SNACKS

NOTES & REMINDERS

DOODLE MY MOOD

BREAKFAST IDEAS

LUNCH IDEAS

DINNER IDEAS

STAYING *On Track*

MY WEIGHT LOSS DIARY:

_____

_____

_____

_____

WATER TRACKER

○ ○ ○ ○ ○ ○ ○

LOW CARB SNACKS

NOTES & REMINDERS

_____

_____

_____

_____

_____

_____

_____

_____

_____

DOODLE MY MOOD

BREAKFAST IDEAS

LUNCH IDEAS

DINNER IDEAS

STAYING *On Track*

MY WEIGHT LOSS DIARY:

WATER TRACKER

LOW CARB SNACKS

NOTES & REMINDERS

DOODLE MY MOOD

BREAKFAST IDEAS

LUNCH IDEAS

DINNER IDEAS

STAYING *On Track*

MY WEIGHT LOSS DIARY:

_____

_____

_____

_____

_____

WATER TRACKER

LOW CARB SNACKS

NOTES & REMINDERS

DOODLE MY MOOD

BREAKFAST IDEAS

LUNCH IDEAS

DINNER IDEAS

STAYING *On Track*

MY WEIGHT LOSS DIARY:

WATER TRACKER

LOW CARB SNACKS

NOTES & REMINDERS

DOODLE MY MOOD

BREAKFAST IDEAS

LUNCH IDEAS

DINNER IDEAS

MEAL *Planner*

GROCERY LIST

☐
☐
☐
☐
☐
☐
☐
☐
☐
☐
☐
☐
☐
☐
☐
☐

MON

TUES

WED

THUR

FRI

SAT

SUN

KETO *Recipe*

RECIPE NAME:

	Keto	Low Carb	Paleo	Vegetarian	Vegan	Dairy Free	Gluten Free
	☐	☐	☐	☐	☐	☐	☐

QTY	INGREDIENTS	RECIPE INSTRUCTIONS

NOTES & RECIPE REVIEW

Serves	
Prep Time	
Cook Time	
Tools	
Temp	

Total	Carbs	Fat	Protein	Cals

DAILY FOOD *Tracker*

FOOD TRACKER

MEAL/SNACK	NET CARBS	FAT	CAL	PROTEIN
DAILY GOAL:				
TOTAL:				

NOTES & MEAL IDEAS

FITNESS TRACKER

		Notes
Type		
Time		
Avg HR		
Max HR		
Reps		
Cals		

DAILY OVERVIEW

		Notes		
Sleep			On Track	
Water Intake				
Steps Taken				
Active Mins			Goal Met	
Active Hours				
Cals Burned				

DAILY FOOD *Tracker*

FOOD TRACKER

MEAL/SNACK	NET CARBS	FAT	CAL	PROTEIN
DAILY GOAL:				
TOTAL:				

NOTES & MEAL IDEAS

FITNESS TRACKER

Type		Notes
Time		
Avg HR		
Max HR		
Reps		
Cals		

DAILY OVERVIEW

Sleep		Notes	On Track
Water Intake			
Steps Taken			
Active Mins			Goal Met
Active Hours			
Cals Burned			

DAILY FOOD *Tracker*

FOOD TRACKER

MEAL/SNACK	NET CARBS	FAT	CAL	PROTEIN
DAILY GOAL:				
TOTAL:				

NOTES & MEAL IDEAS

FITNESS TRACKER

		Notes
Type		
Time		
Avg HR		
Max HR		
Reps		
Cals		

DAILY OVERVIEW

		Notes		
Sleep			On Track	
Water Intake				
Steps Taken				
Active Mins			Goal Met	
Active Hours				
Cals Burned				

DAILY FOOD *Tracker*

FOOD TRACKER

MEAL/SNACK	NET CARBS	FAT	CAL	PROTEIN
DAILY GOAL:				
TOTAL:				

NOTES & MEAL IDEAS

FITNESS TRACKER

		Notes
Type		
Time		
Avg HR		
Max HR		
Reps		
Cals		

DAILY OVERVIEW

		Notes		On Track
Sleep				
Water Intake				
Steps Taken				
Active Mins				Goal Met
Active Hours				
Cals Burned				

DAILY FOOD *Tracker*

FOOD TRACKER

MEAL/SNACK	NET CARBS	FAT	CAL	PROTEIN
DAILY GOAL:				
TOTAL:				

NOTES & MEAL IDEAS

FITNESS TRACKER

Type		Notes
Time		
Avg HR		
Max HR		
Reps		
Cals		

DAILY OVERVIEW

Sleep		Notes		On Track
Water Intake				
Steps Taken				
Active Mins				Goal Met
Active Hours				
Cals Burned				

DAILY FOOD *Tracker*

FOOD TRACKER

MEAL/SNACK	NET CARBS	FAT	CAL	PROTEIN
DAILY GOAL:				
TOTAL:				

NOTES & MEAL IDEAS

FITNESS TRACKER

Type		Notes
Time		
Avg HR		
Max HR		
Reps		
Cals		

DAILY OVERVIEW

Sleep		Notes		On Track
Water Intake				
Steps Taken				
Active Mins				Goal Met
Active Hours				
Cals Burned				

DAILY FOOD *Tracker*

FOOD TRACKER

MEAL/SNACK	NET CARBS	FAT	CAL	PROTEIN
DAILY GOAL:				
TOTAL:				

NOTES & MEAL IDEAS

FITNESS TRACKER

Type		Notes
Time		
Avg HR		
Max HR		
Reps		
Cals		

DAILY OVERVIEW

Sleep		Notes		On Track
Water Intake				
Steps Taken				
Active Mins				Goal Met
Active Hours				
Cals Burned				

KETO GO TO *Meals*

FAVORITE KETO FRIENDLY MEALS

BREAKFAST	LUNCH	DINNER	SNACKS
BREAKFAST	LUNCH	DINNER	SNACKS
BREAKFAST	LUNCH	DINNER	SNACKS
BREAKFAST	LUNCH	DINNER	SNACKS
BREAKFAST	LUNCH	DINNER	SNACKS
BREAKFAST	LUNCH	DINNER	SNACKS
BREAKFAST	LUNCH	DINNER	SNACKS

12 WEEK *Keto Meal Tracker*

12 Week Keto Challenge

MONTH	JAN	FEB	MAR	APR	MAY	JUN	JUL	AUG	SEP	OCT	NOV	DEC
WEEK	01	02	03	04	05	06	07	08	09	10	11	12

	BREAKFAST	LUNCH	DINNER	SNACKS
M				
T				
W				
T				
F				
S				
S				

GROCERY SHOPPING LIST / RECIPE INGREDIENTS

WEIGHT LOSS *Journal*

MONDAY

TUESDAY

WEDNESDAY

THURSDAY

FRIDAY

SATURDAY

SUNDAY

WEEK OF:

DATE	WEIGHT LOSS ACTION PLAN

NOTES

WEIGHT LOSS *Tracker*

MONTHLY GOAL

DATE:

	BUST				
	WAIST				
	HIPS				
	BICEP				
	THIGH				
	CALF				
	WEIGHT				

TOTAL WEIGHT LOSS >>

MONTHLY PROGRESS *Tracker*

JAN   FEB   MAR   APR   MAY   JUN   JUL   AUG   SEP   OCT   NOV   DEC

MON	TUE	WED	THU	FRI	SAT	SUN

WEIGHT LOSS MILESTONE TRACKER

CHEAT DAY TRACKER

WEEKLY DIET SUCCESS TRACKER & NOTES

MY WEIGHT LOSS *Routine*

CREATING A ROUTINE FOR SUCCESS

WEIGHT LOSS SUCCESS: HABIT & ROUTINE TRACKER	
DRINK LOTS OF WATER TODAY	**TRACK TOTAL CARB INTAKE**

COMPLETE TOP 3 GOALS OF THE DAY

1
2
3

PLAN MY MEALS FOR THE DAY:

BREAKFAST	LUNCH	DINNER

DAILY TRACKER & TO DO LIST	ACCOMPLISHMENTS

NOTES

WEEKLY *Fasting Tracker*

Week Of: _____

MONDAY

Goal	12	1	2	3	4	5	6	7	8	9	10	11	12	1	2	3	4	5	6	7	8	9	10	11
Actual	12	1	2	3	4	5	6	7	8	9	10	11	12	1	2	3	4	5	6	7	8	9	10	11

TUESDAY

Goal	12	1	2	3	4	5	6	7	8	9	10	11	12	1	2	3	4	5	6	7	8	9	10	11
Actual	12	1	2	3	4	5	6	7	8	9	10	11	12	1	2	3	4	5	6	7	8	9	10	11

WEDNESDAY

Goal	12	1	2	3	4	5	6	7	8	9	10	11	12	1	2	3	4	5	6	7	8	9	10	11
Actual	12	1	2	3	4	5	6	7	8	9	10	11	12	1	2	3	4	5	6	7	8	9	10	11

THURSDAY

Goal	12	1	2	3	4	5	6	7	8	9	10	11	12	1	2	3	4	5	6	7	8	9	10	11
Actual	12	1	2	3	4	5	6	7	8	9	10	11	12	1	2	3	4	5	6	7	8	9	10	11

FRIDAY

Goal	12	1	2	3	4	5	6	7	8	9	10	11	12	1	2	3	4	5	6	7	8	9	10	11
Actual	12	1	2	3	4	5	6	7	8	9	10	11	12	1	2	3	4	5	6	7	8	9	10	11

SATURDAY

Goal	12	1	2	3	4	5	6	7	8	9	10	11	12	1	2	3	4	5	6	7	8	9	10	11
Actual	12	1	2	3	4	5	6	7	8	9	10	11	12	1	2	3	4	5	6	7	8	9	10	11

SUNDAY

Goal	12	1	2	3	4	5	6	7	8	9	10	11	12	1	2	3	4	5	6	7	8	9	10	11
Actual	12	1	2	3	4	5	6	7	8	9	10	11	12	1	2	3	4	5	6	7	8	9	10	11

WEEK OF: _____

KETO *Meal* LOG BOOK

	BREAKFAST	LUNCH	DINNER	SNACKS
MONDAY				
TUESDAY				
WEDNESDAY				
THURSDAY				
FRIDAY				
SATURDAY				
SUNDAY				

MY PROGRESS *Tracker*

SLEEP TRACKER:

DATE

☀ RISE: | 🌙 BEDTIME: | 💭 SLEEP (HRS):

NOTES FOR THE DAY

IN A STATE OF KETOSIS?

YES   NO   UNSURE

WATER INTAKE TRACKER

EXERCISE / WORKOUT ROUTINE

DAILY ENERGY LEVEL		
HIGH	**MEDIUM**	**LOW**

BREAKFAST

FAT: CARBS: PROTEIN: CALORIES:

LUNCH

FAT: CARBS: PROTEIN: CALORIES:

DINNER

FAT: CARBS: PROTEIN: CALORIES:

SNACKS

FAT: CARBS: PROTEIN: CALORIES:

TOP 6 PRIORITIES OF THE DAY

END OF THE DAY TOTAL OVERVIEW

CARBS   FAT   PROTEIN   CALORIES

Macro Quick Reference

MACRO TRACKER

QTY	TYPE	PROTEIN	FAT	CARBS	CALS	NOTES

INTERMITTENT *Fasting Log*

WEEK OF:

	START TIME	END TIME	TOTAL FAST HRS
M	:	:	:
T	:	:	:
W	:	:	:
T	:	:	:
F	:	:	:
S	:	:	:
S	:	:	:

WEEK OF:

	START TIME	END TIME	TOTAL FAST HRS
M	:	:	:
T	:	:	:
W	:	:	:
T	:	:	:
F	:	:	:
S	:	:	:
S	:	:	:

WEEK OF:

	START TIME	END TIME	TOTAL FAST HRS
M	:	:	:
T	:	:	:
W	:	:	:
T	:	:	:
F	:	:	:
S	:	:	:
S	:	:	:

WEEK OF:

	START TIME	END TIME	TOTAL FAST HRS
M	:	:	:
T	:	:	:
W	:	:	:
T	:	:	:
F	:	:	:
S	:	:	:
S	:	:	:

WEEK OF:

	START TIME	END TIME	TOTAL FAST HRS
M	:	:	:
T	:	:	:
W	:	:	:
T	:	:	:
F	:	:	:
S	:	:	:
S	:	:	:

WEEK OF:

	START TIME	END TIME	TOTAL FAST HRS
M	:	:	:
T	:	:	:
W	:	:	:
T	:	:	:
F	:	:	:
S	:	:	:
S	:	:	:

MILESTONES & ACCOMPLISHMENTS

NOTES & REFLECTIONS

GOALS & *Accomplishments*

MONTH | JAN FEB MAR APR MAY JUN JUL AUG SEP OCT NOV DEC

THIS MONTH'S **GOALS**

ACTION PLAN

M T W T F S S

NOTES:

WEEKLY GOALS

M

T

W

T

F

S

S

THOUGHTS

MEALS:	BREAKFAST	LUNCH	DINNER	SNACKS
M				
T				
W				
T				
F				
S				
S				

Low Carb Shopping List

FRESH PRODUCE

MEAT AND SEAFOOD

DAIRY PRODUCTS

PANTRY ITEMS

FROZEN / OTHER

Keto Friendly Foods

KETO FRIENDLY FOODS	NET CARBS	PROTEINS	FAT

FOODS TO EAT IN MODERATION	NET CARBS	PROTEINS	FAT

STAYING *On Track*

MY WEIGHT LOSS DIARY:

WATER TRACKER

LOW CARB SNACKS

NOTES & REMINDERS

DOODLE MY MOOD

BREAKFAST IDEAS

LUNCH IDEAS

DINNER IDEAS

STAYING *On Track*

MY WEIGHT LOSS DIARY:

_____

_____

_____

_____

WATER TRACKER

NOTES & REMINDERS

DOODLE MY MOOD

LOW CARB SNACKS

BREAKFAST IDEAS

LUNCH IDEAS

DINNER IDEAS

STAYING *On Track*

MY WEIGHT LOSS DIARY:

WATER TRACKER

LOW CARB SNACKS

NOTES & REMINDERS

DOODLE MY MOOD

BREAKFAST IDEAS

LUNCH IDEAS

DINNER IDEAS

STAYING *On Track*

MY WEIGHT LOSS DIARY:

_____
_____
_____
_____

WATER TRACKER

NOTES & REMINDERS

DOODLE MY MOOD

LOW CARB SNACKS

BREAKFAST IDEAS

LUNCH IDEAS

DINNER IDEAS

STAYING *On Track*

MY WEIGHT LOSS DIARY:

WATER TRACKER

LOW CARB SNACKS

NOTES & REMINDERS

DOODLE MY MOOD

BREAKFAST IDEAS

LUNCH IDEAS

DINNER IDEAS

STAYING *On Track*

MY WEIGHT LOSS DIARY:

_____

_____

_____

_____

WATER TRACKER

LOW CARB SNACKS

NOTES & REMINDERS

DOODLE MY MOOD

BREAKFAST IDEAS

LUNCH IDEAS

DINNER IDEAS

STAYING *On Track*

MY WEIGHT LOSS DIARY:

WATER TRACKER

NOTES & REMINDERS

DOODLE MY MOOD

LOW CARB SNACKS

BREAKFAST IDEAS

LUNCH IDEAS

DINNER IDEAS

MEAL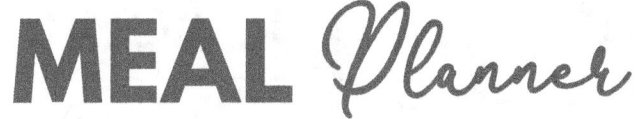

WEEK OF

GROCERY LIST

☐
☐
☐
☐
☐
☐
☐
☐
☐
☐
☐
☐
☐
☐
☐
☐
☐
☐

MON

TUES

WED

THUR

FRI

SAT

SUN

WEEK OF:

KETO *Meal* LOG BOOK

	BREAKFAST	LUNCH	DINNER	SNACKS
MONDAY				
TUESDAY				
WEDNESDAY				
THURSDAY				
FRIDAY				
SATURDAY				
SUNDAY				

WEEKLY *Fasting Tracker*

Week Of: _____

MONDAY

	12	1	2	3	4	5	6	7	8	9	10	11	12	1	2	3	4	5	6	7	8	9	10	11
Goal	12	1	2	3	4	5	6	7	8	9	10	11	12	1	2	3	4	5	6	7	8	9	10	11
Actual	12	1	2	3	4	5	6	7	8	9	10	11	12	1	2	3	4	5	6	7	8	9	10	11

TUESDAY

	12	1	2	3	4	5	6	7	8	9	10	11	12	1	2	3	4	5	6	7	8	9	10	11
Goal	12	1	2	3	4	5	6	7	8	9	10	11	12	1	2	3	4	5	6	7	8	9	10	11
Actual	12	1	2	3	4	5	6	7	8	9	10	11	12	1	2	3	4	5	6	7	8	9	10	11

WEDNESDAY

	12	1	2	3	4	5	6	7	8	9	10	11	12	1	2	3	4	5	6	7	8	9	10	11
Goal	12	1	2	3	4	5	6	7	8	9	10	11	12	1	2	3	4	5	6	7	8	9	10	11
Actual	12	1	2	3	4	5	6	7	8	9	10	11	12	1	2	3	4	5	6	7	8	9	10	11

THURSDAY

	12	1	2	3	4	5	6	7	8	9	10	11	12	1	2	3	4	5	6	7	8	9	10	11
Goal	12	1	2	3	4	5	6	7	8	9	10	11	12	1	2	3	4	5	6	7	8	9	10	11
Actual	12	1	2	3	4	5	6	7	8	9	10	11	12	1	2	3	4	5	6	7	8	9	10	11

FRIDAY

	12	1	2	3	4	5	6	7	8	9	10	11	12	1	2	3	4	5	6	7	8	9	10	11
Goal	12	1	2	3	4	5	6	7	8	9	10	11	12	1	2	3	4	5	6	7	8	9	10	11
Actual	12	1	2	3	4	5	6	7	8	9	10	11	12	1	2	3	4	5	6	7	8	9	10	11

SATURDAY

	12	1	2	3	4	5	6	7	8	9	10	11	12	1	2	3	4	5	6	7	8	9	10	11
Goal	12	1	2	3	4	5	6	7	8	9	10	11	12	1	2	3	4	5	6	7	8	9	10	11
Actual	12	1	2	3	4	5	6	7	8	9	10	11	12	1	2	3	4	5	6	7	8	9	10	11

SUNDAY

	12	1	2	3	4	5	6	7	8	9	10	11	12	1	2	3	4	5	6	7	8	9	10	11
Goal	12	1	2	3	4	5	6	7	8	9	10	11	12	1	2	3	4	5	6	7	8	9	10	11
Actual	12	1	2	3	4	5	6	7	8	9	10	11	12	1	2	3	4	5	6	7	8	9	10	11

Weekly Meal Planner

Week of: _____

	Breakfast	Lunch	Dinner	Snack	Other
Monday	TOTAL Carbs Fat Protein Cals	TOTAL Carbs Fat Protein Cals	TOTAL Carbs Fat Protein Cals	TOTAL Carbs Fat Protein Cals	TOTAL Carbs Fat Protein Cals
Tuesday	TOTAL Carbs Fat Protein Cals	TOTAL Carbs Fat Protein Cals	TOTAL Carbs Fat Protein Cals	TOTAL Carbs Fat Protein Cals	TOTAL Carbs Fat Protein Cals
Wednesday	TOTAL Carbs Fat Protein Cals	TOTAL Carbs Fat Protein Cals	TOTAL Carbs Fat Protein Cals	TOTAL Carbs Fat Protein Cals	TOTAL Carbs Fat Protein Cals
Thursday	TOTAL Carbs Fat Protein Cals	TOTAL Carbs Fat Protein Cals	TOTAL Carbs Fat Protein Cals	TOTAL Carbs Fat Protein Cals	TOTAL Carbs Fat Protein Cals
Friday	TOTAL Carbs Fat Protein Cals	TOTAL Carbs Fat Protein Cals	TOTAL Carbs Fat Protein Cals	TOTAL Carbs Fat Protein Cals	TOTAL Carbs Fat Protein Cals
Saturday	TOTAL Carbs Fat Protein Cals	TOTAL Carbs Fat Protein Cals	TOTAL Carbs Fat Protein Cals	TOTAL Carbs Fat Protein Cals	TOTAL Carbs Fat Protein Cals
Sunday	TOTAL Carbs Fat Protein Cals	TOTAL Carbs Fat Protein Cals	TOTAL Carbs Fat Protein Cals	TOTAL Carbs Fat Protein Cals	TOTAL Carbs Fat Protein Cals

WEIGHT LOSS *Journal*

MONDAY

TUESDAY

WEDNESDAY

THURSDAY

FRIDAY

SATURDAY

SUNDAY

WEEK OF:

DATE	WEIGHT LOSS ACTION PLAN

NOTES

WEIGHT LOSS *Tracker*

WEEKLY WEIGHT LOSS TRACKER

MONTHLY GOAL

DATE:

BUST					
WAIST					
HIPS					
BICEP					
THIGH					
CALF					
WEIGHT					

TOTAL WEIGHT LOSS >>